Bodyweight Training for Martial Arts
By Matt Schifferle

Text Copyright © 2019 Matthew J. Schifferle
All Rights Reserved

ISBN- 9781093665703

The information provided in this book is designed to provide helpful information on the subjects discussed. This book is not meant to be used, nor should it be used, to diagnose or treat any medical condition. For diagnosis or treatment of any medical problem, consult your physician. The publisher and author are not responsible for any specific health or allergy needs that may require medical supervision and are not liable for any damages or negative consequences from any treatment, action, application or preparation, to any person reading or following the information in this book. References are provided for informational purposes only and do not constitute endorsement of any websites or other sources. Readers should be aware that the websites listed in this book may change.

Cover photo and design by Chris Clemens at http://www.thinkpilgrim.com

Dedicated to David Crowe,
and the high kicking students at Kojo Academy of Taekwon-Do.

Table of Contents

Introduction	5
Chapter 1 The Advantages of Calisthenics for Martial Arts Conditioning	7
Chapter 2 Four Training Methods For Complete Martial Arts Conditioning	13
Chapter 3 How to Develop Supreme Punching Power With Push-Ups	18
Chapter 4 Developing Pulling Strength With Rows	35
Chapter 5 Building Rock-Solid Legs	50
Chapter 6 Build Punch-Proof Abs With Leg Raises	65
Chapter 7 Accessory Exercises to Strengthen Weak Links	77
Chapter 8 Routines for Success	85
Chapter 9 How to Be Action-Ready At All Times	114

Introduction

Welcome to Bodyweight Training for Martial Arts! The exercises and strategies in this book will teach you how to develop the physical qualities you need to perform at your best as a martial artist. Whether you're in MMA, Jiu-Jitsu, Karate, or even Tai-Chi these holistic and practical exercises will take your training to the next level and beyond.

Who the heck am I?

My name is Matt Schifferle, and I've been a martial artist since age ten. Over the years, I've used a wide range of conditioning methods, from classic bodybuilding programs to wearing weights while kicking. Everything worked to at least some degree, but all methods also came with a high price to pay. Some workouts took up so much time and energy that I had little left for my martial arts classes. Other approaches left me feeling slow and stiff. A few methods even threatened my entire martial arts career with muscle imbalances and injury. Everything always felt like one step forward and one step back.

The more I tried to get in top shape, the more frustrated I became. Martial arts were my gateway to physical training. It was how I learned the value of using a disciplined mind to transform my body. Now, here I was feeling like my gym workouts were putting my martial arts training in jeopardy.

After nearly 20 years of lifting iron, I was beat up, fed up, and ready to give up. Not just on exercise, but even my Taekwon-Do. Thankfully, I started to learn about a discipline called progressive calisthenics, and my world changed forever. At long last, there was a training method that seemed to be all pros without any cons. Other approaches left me feeling used and abused, but calisthenics made me strong and resilient. As I write this, I've been practicing martial arts for 31 years and calisthenics for 10. Never before have I felt this strong, limber, and explosive while also remaining free of stiffness and joint pain. I'm in better shape and a better martial artist, now at age 41 than when I was in my 20s!

My story is not that unusual. I've shared what I've learned through my Red Delta Project and have heard from many who've had a similar experience. Men and women who once thought they were past their prime as martial artists have infused new life into their training with just a few simple calisthenics drills.

I attribute much of my success to the influence martial arts have had on my mind and body. Now it's my chance to pay it forward and present you with this book. The information within these pages can quite possibly enhance your martial arts training beyond anything you believe is possible. It may even save your training career. I know it certainly saved mine, and for that, I'm ever thankful.

Keep kicking,

-Matt Schifferle

Chapter 1

The Advantages of Calisthenics for Martial Arts Conditioning

Bodyweight exercise and martial arts have been training partners ever since people learned how to throw a punch. Some of the oldest fighting styles have traditionally included calisthenics training as part of the regular training routine.

One of the best examples of this is the traditional Shaolin training system. When you observe the classic styles, it's hard to draw a definitive line between calisthenics and martial arts. Legend has it the Shaolin fighting systems were developed from the calisthenics the monks were using to condition themselves for long hours of meditation.

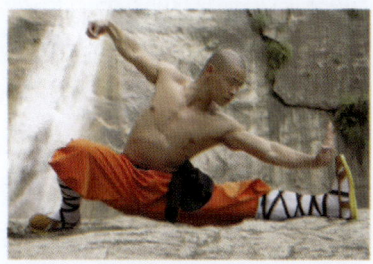

A classic style practiced by a modern warrior shows how calisthenics and martial arts share a rich history. Photo: Ancient-origins.net

Such physical conditioning sure wasn't restricted to the far east. In Europe, physical conditioning was required training to become a formidable fighter from the Knights of medieval Europe to ancient Greece's wrestling styles. Once again, training to fight and training to be athletically capable were considered the same. After all, how can someone be a proficient fighter if they can't skillfully use their body? At the same time, you could argue that someone wouldn't have a complete physical fitness level if they couldn't fight and defend themselves.

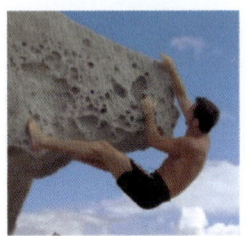 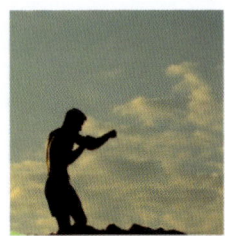 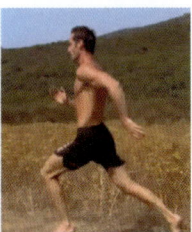

The Movnat organization includes various disciplines, including climbing, running, crawling, swimming, and basic martial arts techniques. Photo: Images from the Movnat promotional video on movnat.com.

The three risks modern conditioning poses to your martial arts proficiency

Despite the long synergistic history of conditioning and martial arts training, the two disciplines have been practiced separately for the past few generations. Some experts have even criticized the idea of spending valuable energy at the gym instead of practicing kicks and sparring. Growing up, I remember my instructors advising me to avoid strength training because it would make me tight and slow.

It's easy to scoff at an idea like that now, but it's not entirely without merit. Strength training can pose several risks to your martial arts proficiency. One such risk is the interference effect; when you spend so much effort in the gym, it starts to impede upon your martial arts training. I've seen this happen to several people who often boast about how hard they work out but later claim they feel sluggish and tired in the Dojo.

The second challenge is the risk of injury. It's a shame when poor lifting technique or excessive loads hurt both your body and your martial arts practice. Sometimes, these injuries can be acute and happen suddenly, but most issues creep up over time and can take months to identify and resolve. That's a long time to suffer through compromised martial arts training, especially if you're preparing for a competition.

The last significant risk of inappropriate conditioning is the lack of functional carryover. In exercise physiology, there's something known as the S.A.I.D principle, which stands for specific adaptation to imposed demand. It means that all exercises develop the unique physical qualities required by that same activity in simple terms. This training principle is why you'll never become a world-class hockey player even if you're an Olympic figure skater, or an elite sprinter no matter how many marathons you complete. There is, however, a degree of functional carryover where some of the functional abilities overlap. The figure skater may not have a good slap shot but can probably learn how to skate like a hockey player pretty quickly since they are already comfortable on the ice.

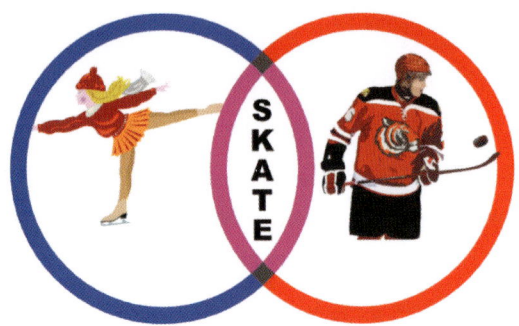

Functional carryover depends on how someone may apply the functional demands of one activity to another.

Supplemental conditioning will only improve your performance if there's an appropriate amount of functional carryover between it and your sport.

For example, you'll find that squats and lunges may have a lot of functional carryover to jumping because both exercises use your legs in similar ways. Meanwhile, you may find some activities have minimal functional carryover to your martial arts practice because of the lack of similarity.

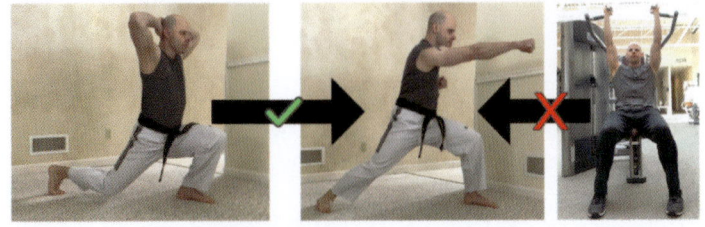

The lunge exercise has many functional similarities to martial arts applications, while using a stabilized weight machine may have minimal functional carryover.

Recognizing these risks can help us understand how some experts may believe physical conditioning could be detrimental to one's martial arts performance. Spending too much energy on risky exercises that have limited functional carryover can indeed hold anyone back.

The calisthenics solution

The ideal martial arts conditioning program should minimize all three of these risks. You want a method that requires few resources while making you physically and mentally resilient and contains as much functional carryover as possible.

These are the reasons why bodyweight training is such a perfect fit for any disciplined martial artist. Its practical nature means you don't need to visit a gym to practice lengthy and costly workout routines. You can even get in a few sets while warming up for a class or keep your skills sharp while traveling.

When practiced correctly, bodyweight training places less stress on the joints and nervous system. There is less wear and tear on your body without leaving you exhausted and drained for practice.

Lastly, calisthenics is a highly functional discipline. The primary goal of calisthenics is to learn how to use your own body better. Sure, you'll become more proficient in exercises like push-ups and lunges, but that proficiency comes from building more than just strength. You'll also develop qualities like stability, mobility, and the coordinated use of your muscles. Achieving this higher level of self-understanding is the key to maximizing your functional carryover.

It's certainly possible to achieve these benefits with other training methods, but it's hard to find all of these qualities in one efficient discipline like calisthenics. Simply put, bodyweight training will bring you the most benefit with the lowest cost to your martial arts training and lifestyle. I could write a whole book on the benefits of calisthenics training, but I would rather show you so you can experience them for yourself. Let's get right to it and explore the most effective training methods for martial arts training.

Chapter 2

4 Training Methods For Complete Martial Arts Conditioning

One of the biggest mistakes martial artists make in their conditioning is they only train a very narrow range of physical performance. As a martial artist, your body is a versatile multi-tool. You use your muscles to perform a massive range of capabilities and functional attributes.

The wide range of functional requirements in martial arts is why this book doesn't use just one way to perform basic calisthenics exercises. The four methods covered in this book won't leave you with just a lot of stationary strength while neglecting your stability and mobility. They also won't give you a lot of isometric strength while robbing you of explosive power. Here are the four basic approaches to complete martial arts conditioning.

#1 Technical progressions

Bodyweight training is a discipline you progress through technical adjustment. Whereas with weightlifting, you maintain your technique and adjust the load you lift, bodyweight training is the opposite. Your weight stays consistent while you change your technique.

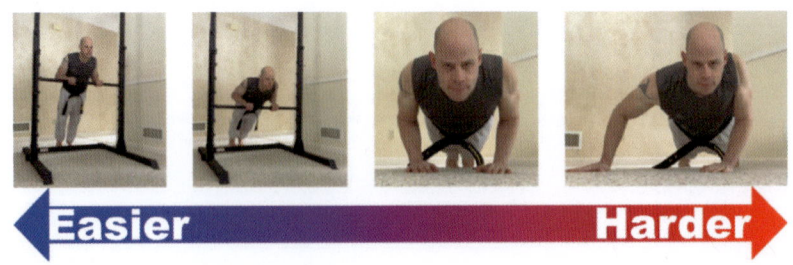

The progressive technical aspect of bodyweight training is sometimes perceived as a disadvantage as many people believe it's easier to add weight to an exercise to progress. In some respects, this is true, but there's a massive advantage to using a technical progression, especially in martial arts.

Technical progression develops all three of the functional qualities you need to perform at your best. These basic progressions will ensure you'll build strength, mobility, and stability for complete physiological preparation. Better yet, you'll be developing these qualities within just a few exercises. You won't need to invest in a lot of exercises, exhausting workouts, or equipment.

#2 Shifting work

Martial arts training can involve a lot of fluid movements and positions. Even linear striking styles can involve diverse movements, especially when it comes to sparring. Meanwhile, strength training is something you usually practice using bilateral mechanical motions that move along the sagittal plane.

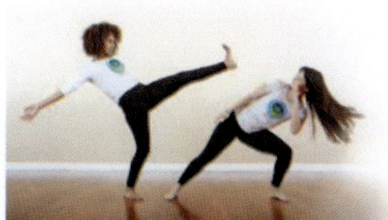

Martial arts require strength and stability in all three dimensions of space, as these two Capoeira students demonstrate. Photo: SeattleCapoeiraCenter.com

This practical challenge is why I included what I call shift work in this program. Shift work helps you break out of the straight up and down linear conditioning patterns and enables you to build a broader "foundation of strength." This sort of training also teaches your muscles to be strong, mobile, and stable while performing unstable movements. You'll build not only a more resilient body but also the ability to be strong and powerful in almost any physically demanding scenario.

#3 Isometric work

Using strength to move through space is one thing; creating muscle tension to maintain a position is quite another. Most any martial artist has experienced the mental and physical challenge of holding a deep stance or difficult hold for time. This training is very hard, but it's also beneficial for conditioning your muscles to stay strong against an immovable force.

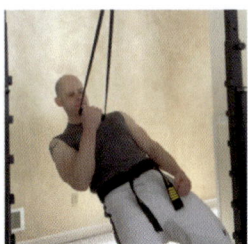 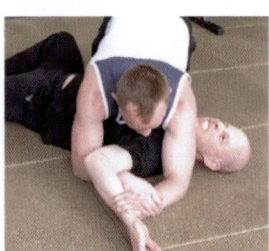

Isometrics are very useful for training your muscles to work against another object, like your opponent.

#4 Explosive work

At the other end of the speed spectrum is the ability to move as fast as possible with explosive training. Using a fast motion in your basic exercises will help you develop the power and control necessary to launch yourself through space.

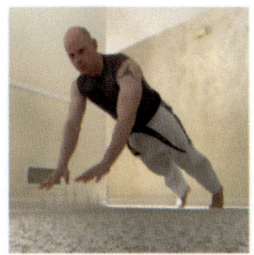 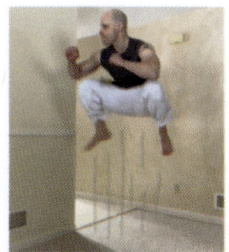

Moving quickly is critical for conditioning speed and power.

So there you have it, the four training methods for complete martial arts strength and conditioning. I like to use the following diagram to illustrate how they all relate to each other.

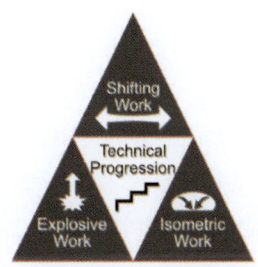

In the center are the primary technical progressions for the basic exercises in this book. Its central location represents that the other three methods can use any technical sequences to adjust the technical difficulty. On the bottom are the isometric and explosive work methods representing the opposite ends of the speed spectrum. At the top, you'll find the shifting work to complete the holistic approach to martial arts conditioning. Each method is one part of the whole, covering everything you need to perform at your best.

Chapter 3

How to Develop Supreme Punching Power With Push-Ups

Few moves have as much functional carryover as the humble push-up. Aside from resembling a punching motion, push-ups also teach you hand strength, shoulder stability, and how to use your whole body behind your fist.

Sadly, few people learn just how practical push-up training can be. Many barely scratch the surface with a couple of half-hearted push-up variations they learned in the Dojo or back in gym class. It's a good start, but there's so much more benefit you can gain from the exercise.
Starting today, you'll venture down the path to earning your black belt in push-ups and more punching power than ever!

Key technical points

The following technical details will make a big difference in the quality of your push-up training.

#1 Avoid weighting the outside of your hands.

Do your best to prevent your hands from "tenting" on the floor or bar. This hand position occurs when you have too much weight on the outside of your hands, causing the thumb and pointer finger to lift. Maintaining weight on the inside of your hand will drive more tension to your working muscles while preventing excessive stress on the wrist, elbow, and shoulder joints.

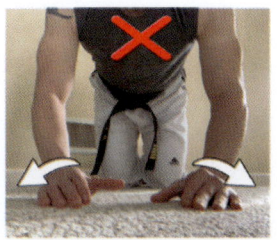 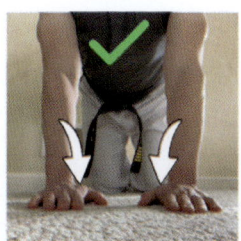

Keeping the weight on the inside of your hands prevents "tenting" and joint stress.

#2 Tuck in your elbows

Most punches don't move the elbows flaring out to the side, so why do push-ups like that? It's much more effective and safer on the joints to keep your elbows in tight to your sides, just like during a punch.

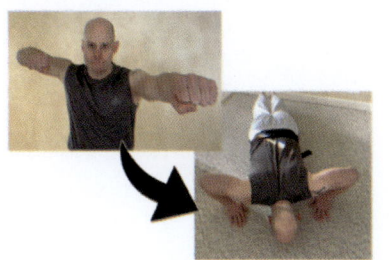 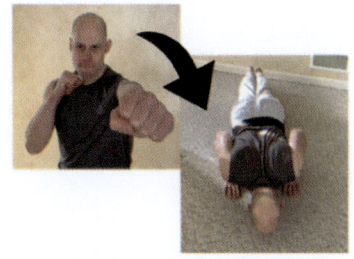

As you punch, so shall you push!

19

#3 Keep your abs, glutes, and back tense

Your punching power is only as strong as the power you can drive to the floor. Be sure to keep your glutes, abs, and quads tense during the push-up to improve body control and tension transition. Maintaining tension in your whole back will improve your shoulder stability and total body strength.

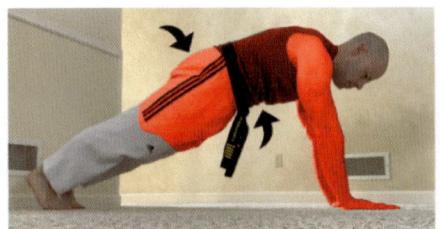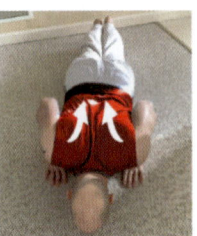

A little extra tension in the glutes, abs, and back goes a long way toward stronger push-ups and punches.

#4 Tense your lower arm and hand

Weak and stiff wrists are a common lament among push-up practitioners and martial artists alike. Some resort to using push-up handles, but these only serve as a temporary crutch and don't fix the real problem. Keeping your forearm tense and slightly "clawing" your fingers into the floor will make your wrists strong enough to handle anything.

Push-up progressions

White Belt- Incline Push-Ups

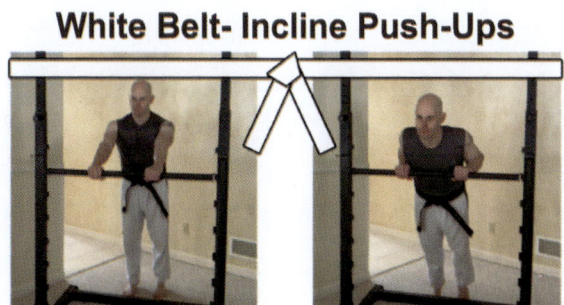

Incline push-ups are a staple exercise for even advanced athletes. Like the basic techniques you learned on your first day in class, no one out-grows this essential exercise.

Inclines are an excellent tool for returning from a long break, improving technique, and warming up. They are also a fun way to practice explosive work as you try to push yourself up into a fully upright position.

The basic rule of progression here is simple, the closer your hands are to the floor, the more resistance you'll put on your muscles. You can find various objects like park benches, countertops, and furniture of multiple heights to measure your progress. If you're in a gym, adjustable height barbell racks or a smith machine are ideal for quantifying your angle to gravity.

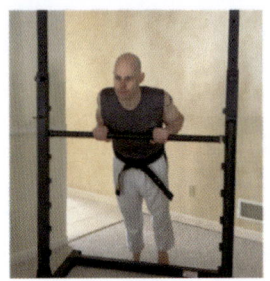 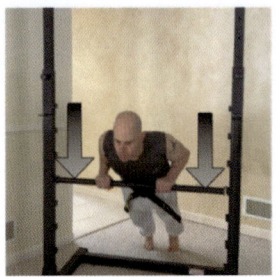

Pushing against a lower support increases the resistance of incline push-ups.

Yellow Belt- Floor Push-Ups

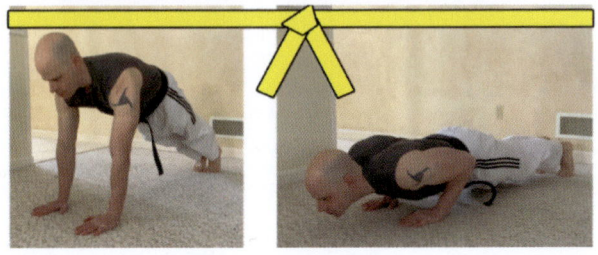

Floor push-ups are about more than just taking your body to the floor. They also incorporate plenty of total body stability and shoulder control plus wrist strength and mobility.

Like incline push-ups, these are a favorite staple for even high-level athletes. Just be sure not to focus too much on this one variation. Too many people make this their main push-up variation while neglecting the benefits of regressive incline push-ups or progressive techniques like close push-ups. They are great to use much of the time, but you don't want to make it the only weapon in your arsenal.

Green Belt- Close Push-Ups

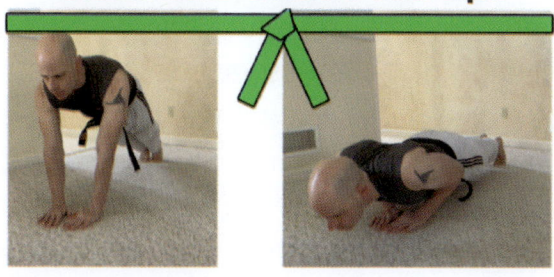

Some athletes call these triceps push-ups, but they are so much more than just extra work for your arm muscles. This variation teaches you how to apply an increasing amount of stability and strength to move your limbs closer to your centerline. This inward pressure helps with punching power, especially when striking out from a close guarded position. It also improves wrist strength and mobility while promoting core control.

Blue Belt- Archer Push-Ups

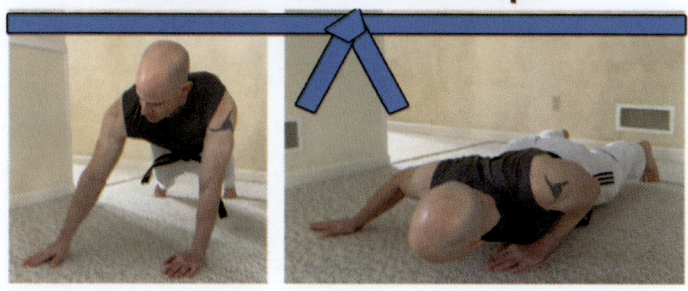

Archer push-ups are like the middle-level belts where you've learned just enough to become dangerous, but the risk is just as much to yourself as anyone else. That's why the demands of the archer push-up are perfect for this stage of your training.

It can be tempting to spread your weight equally between your hands, but try to keep most of your weight on the dominant pressing arm. The further you reach out with the support arm, the more bodyweight you'll load up on the pressing arm.

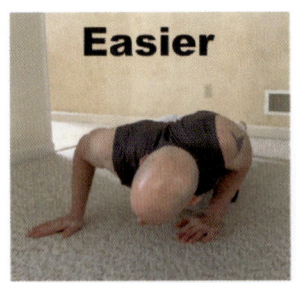
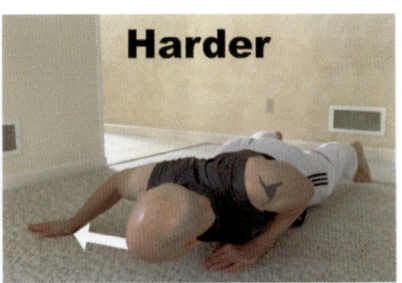

Red Belt- Single-Arm Push-Ups Wide Feet

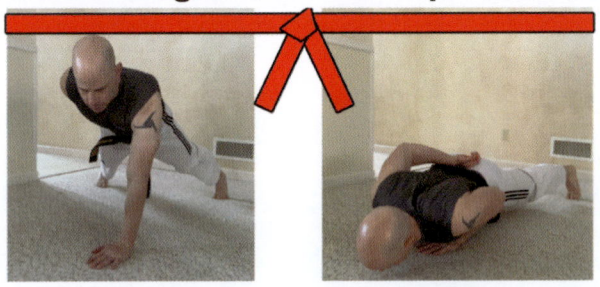

Single-arm push-ups are impressive to witness and even more empowering to practice. They are like the ultimate archer push-up without any support on the other arm at all. Using a wider stance gives you the support you need to deal with the torque generated by your pressing arm. Do your best to keep your pressing hand as close to your centerline as possible to minimize the torque. Yes, that will make the exercise exceedingly more difficult, but that's a good thing, right?

Black Belt- Cobra Push-Ups

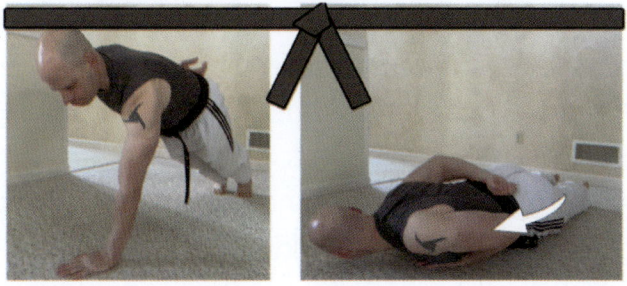

Cobra push-ups are done with your feet close together and bending your body to handle the torque through the torso. This push-up requires a significant amount of strength and total body stability, not to mention coordination that carries over to punching and throwing. Be sure to return to a straight body position at the top of each rep to enforce the dynamic twisting action rather than holding that position throughout the set.

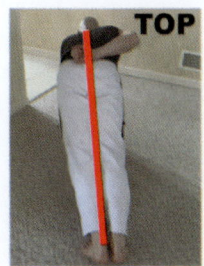 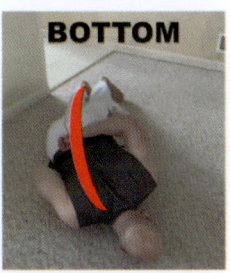

Your torso will want to twist toward the bottom position so let it do as it wants.

Isometric push-ups

Many folks practice push-ups as if they are touching a hot stove. They lower themselves down close to the floor, feel a brief sense of discomfort and then jerk away reflexively. As a result, even long sets of push-ups only engage the muscles at their peak for a few moments.

Isometric push-ups focus directly on the most challenging position in the rep. Instead of jumping out of the hottest point, you're now holding that position for time. This sort of training significantly increases the time under tension at the most challenging point to help you build strength, stability, and mental toughness.

As a general rule, you'll want to hold the lowest position possible with your torso just off the floor. You can decrease the resistance by holding yourself up higher, and this may not be a bad idea on some of the more challenging progressions. Just be sure not to get into a position that allows you to relax into the bottom. Resting at the bottom isn't much of an issue with floor push-ups, but I've seen some athletes settle into a stretched position when using elevated tools like push-up handles.

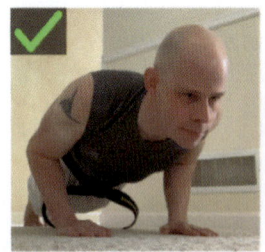 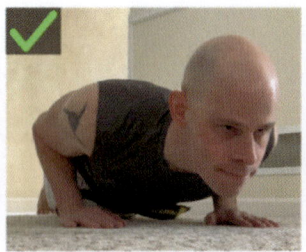 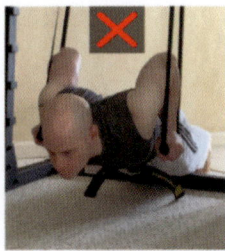

Hold the isometric at any height as long as you don't relax in the bottom position.

Another point to consider is how to get into that bottom position. The most common method is to start at the top and lower yourself into the bottom position, or as low as you can get, and then hold.

The other option is to start on the floor and then slightly lift yourself a couple of inches. I've always preferred this method because it's easier to set the tension throughout your muscles first, and then you can apply resistance after you've set your tension. Lowering yourself down can involve figuring out both the tension and body position simultaneously, which can be more difficult. You can also gradually apply resistance by lifting your torso off the floor while keeping your knees down. Once you've set your tension and position as you want, you raise your knees to apply the full resistance as you maintain your position.

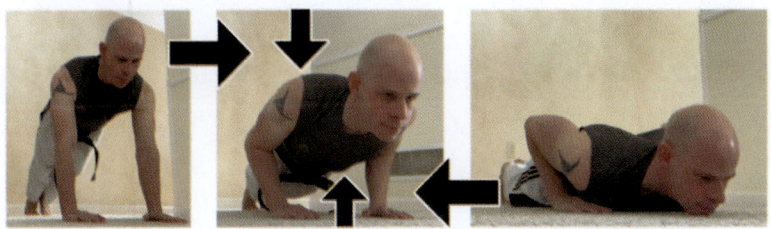

Isometric push-ups can start in the top (left) or bottom (right) position and moving to the point of resistance.

You can also apply this strategy on incline push-ups by assisting yourself with a staggered stance. Once you're in position, then you bring your front foot back to implement the full resistance. When finishing the set, step forward to safely remove the resistance and ease out of the isometric position.

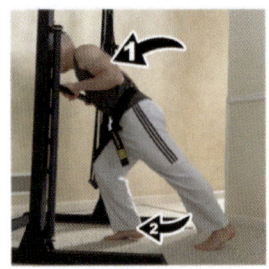 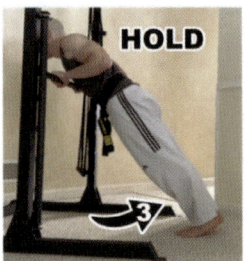 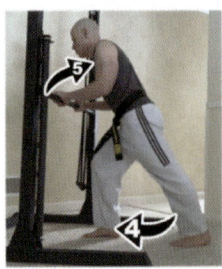

Use one leg to make it easy to get in and out of an incline push-up.

Be sure to keep tension in your whole body, including your chest, shoulders, arms, abs, back, glutes, and legs. You want to make sure your whole body is as stiff as a board and not sagging like a sack of potatoes.

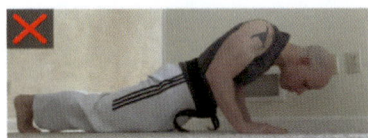 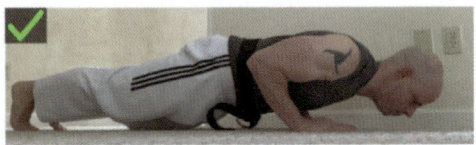

Lastly, maintain smooth and relaxed breathing at all times. It can take some practice to keep your diaphragm relaxed while holding your body tight, but it can help a lot with your endurance on the mat. If you find it difficult to breathe with a particular push-up, regress to an easier technique and practice your breathing with less resistance for a while.

Shifting push-ups

Shifting push-ups are like isometrics where you're controlling your body in an awkward position, only now you're moving from one difficult position to another. Again, this helps you build a broad base of strength and improve your stability in many positions.

Twisting push-ups

Twisting push-ups are a great way to warm up the core and shoulders for a session that may be stressful on the joints. Practice this technique in the bottom position, and gently twist your body while looking to your left and right side. Be sure to do these in a smooth and controlled motion so you don't strain anything. Also, play around with your foot width as some people prefer doing these with their feet close together or about shoulder-width apart.

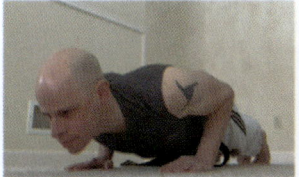 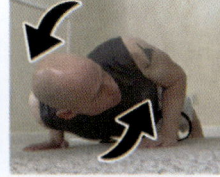 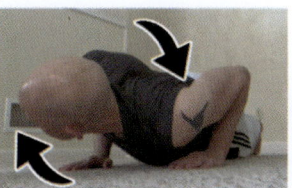

Start Center   **Twist Left**   **Twist Right**

Side to side shifting push-ups

Side-to-side shifting helps build your lateral upper body strength and stability. This motion is similar to archer push-ups only without pressing yourself up off the floor. You can progress this exercise by using a wider hand position where the wider your hands are, the more distance you have to travel while shifting more weight from one arm to another.

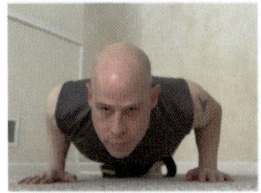 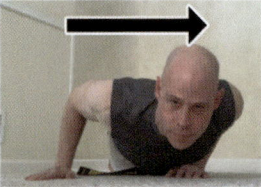 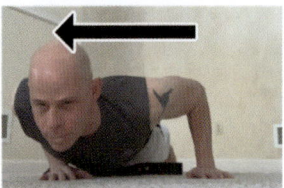

Start Center   **Shift Left**   **Shift Right**

Front and back shifting push-ups

These shifting push-ups are fantastic for improving shoulder stability and wrist mobility, plus they can work your chest muscles like nothing else.

Once again, get down into the bottom position and move your torso forward and back by rocking on the balls of your feet. Pause for 1-3 seconds at the forward and backward position while maintaining tension throughout your whole body.

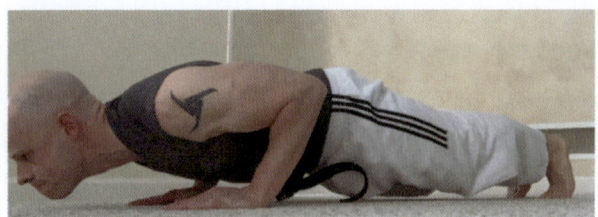

Start Center

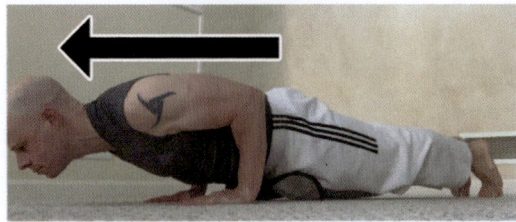

Shift Front

30

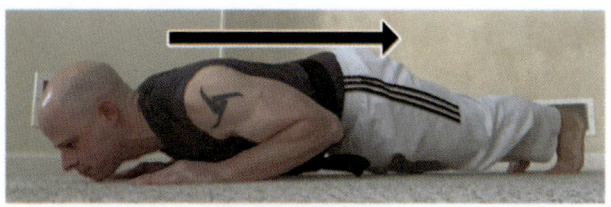

Shift Back

Circular push-ups

These combine all of the shifting push-up variations to create a bit of a wax-on wax-off exercise style. Think of moving your torso in a circular motion along the floor. Be mindful of your wrist mobility and ease into this exercise with small circles at first and progress to bigger circles as your joints and muscles feel ready.

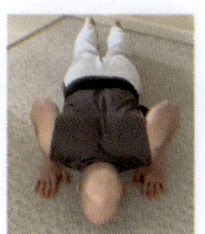 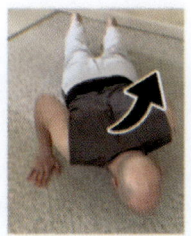 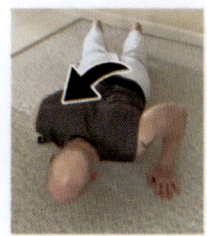 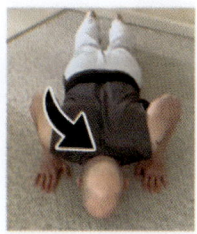

Explosive push-ups

Lastly, we have the explosive push-up. While you can apply an explosive motion to any progression level, most athletes use a standard floor push-up or push-off of an elevated surface. As a word of caution, if you do explosive push-ups on a high surface, like a bar, be extra careful to keep your hands ready to catch you. Otherwise, you may slip and hit yourself on the ledge as you come back down.

The best place to start is to do a push-up with a modest level of resistance. Too much resistance, and you'll not be able to accelerate very well out of the bottom position. Too little, and you won't adequately challenge your nervous system to produce enough power. Pick a variation you can perform 20-30 reps, and that should suit you just fine.

Fast concentric push-ups

The first step of explosive push-up training is to push yourself up with more speed than you would use during your regular push-ups for training strength. Lower yourself into the bottom position, pause a brief second, and then thrust yourself up while maintaining contact with the floor. Pause at the top and repeat.

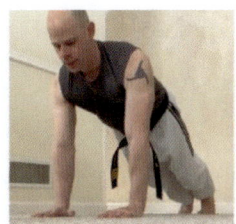
Start at Top

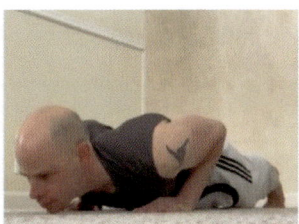
Lower and Pause

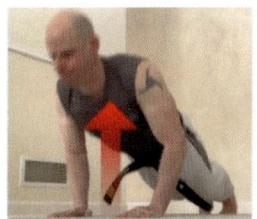
Push Up Fast

Pump reps

The second phase is to do "pump reps," where you eliminate the pause at the top and bottom and lower yourself down in a fast motion. This pace creates a fast pumping tempo similar to what you might use if you're using a bicycle pump or sanding down wood with sandpaper.

Palm raise push-ups

The third phase is to push off the floor with enough force to lift your palms off the floor while your fingers stay touching the ground. This technique creates more pushing power than the first two phases while conditioning your muscles and joints for a soft landing.

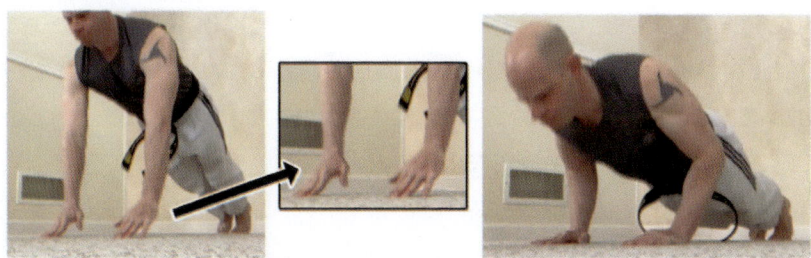

Push hard enough to lift your palms off the floor but maintain contact with your fingers.

Hands off push-ups

This phase is the classic "plyo-push-up." The objective is to push off with so much power that your hands come right off the floor. Once again, be sure to land softly and lower yourself down under control before doing your next rep.

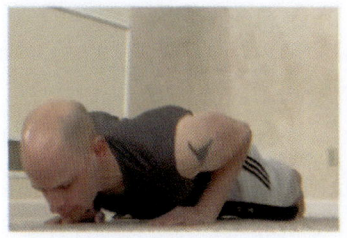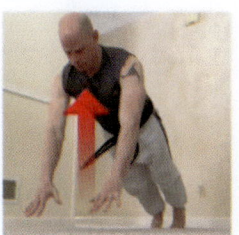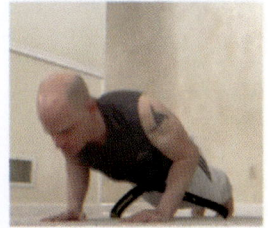

Push off hard enough to jump your hands completely off the floor.

What about clapping hands?

Clapping, slapping, and performing fun acrobatics are very common in the world of explosive push-up training. This stuff is cool, but I've never been a big fan of it myself. I believe it creates an unnecessary risk if you can't get your hands back in position in time for a safe landing. All it takes is just one missed landing to tweak your wrist and compromise your training for a while. That's why I keep my hands under me while doing explosive push-ups. It dramatically reduces the risk of a botched landing, and it doesn't compromise your explosive power in any way.

Chapter 4

Developing Pulling Strength With Rows

Rows always make me think of a game we used to play in a class similar to tug-o-war. We would all pair off, and each of us would place our front foot next to our opponent's front foot. Then, clasping each other's forearm, we would try to pull the other person off balance.

It's a fun game, but I was never very good at it until I learned how to do bodyweight rows. After a few months of progressive rowing, I was surprised by how I could manipulate even heavier opponents with ease. My muscles weren't just stronger; I had also learned how to use my whole body to work as one cohesive unit.

Rows are much more than a general pulling movement. They also require a lot of core and posterior chain stability, which is why I include them in this book. You can generate all the pulling power in the world, but without a stable connection to the ground, all of that power can dissipate.

Key technical points

#1 Twist your arms inward

One of the most common mistakes is to make rowing an arm dominant exercise. Flaring the elbows out without retracting the shoulder blades causes the arms to handle most of the work. That might sound great for building your biceps, but it leaves a lot of strength on the table. Your back muscles are some of the biggest and strongest muscles in your body, and "screwing" your arms into your side will help you tap into their impressive strength.

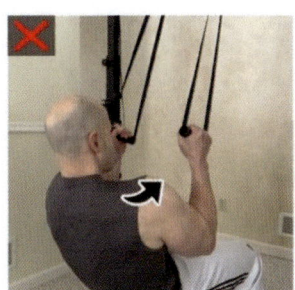 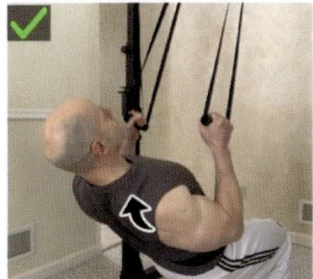

"Screwing" your arm into your shoulder brings more tension to your back and stability in your shoulder joint.

#2 Keep your posterior chain tight

Your pulling strength needs to be grounded to be practical. Keeping every muscle on your backside tense is the best way to improve your stability and power. Concentrate on maintaining tension in your calves, hamstrings, glutes, lower back, and all the muscles up your spine to make your body as stiff as possible.

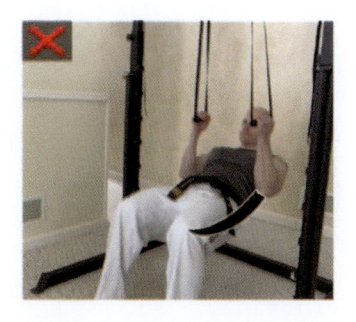

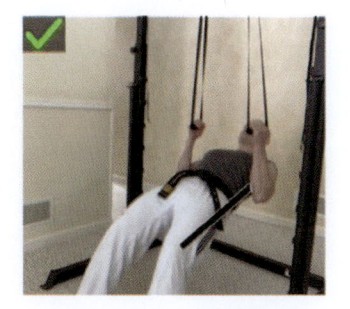

#3 Keep your neck in alignment with your spine

Beware of the tendency to "pigeon" your neck and reach up with your chin. Just like with push-ups, reaching your neck forward can make you feel like you're moving more than you are. Instead, keep your head back so your neck is neutral, and focus on lifting yourself higher by pulling your torso between your hands.

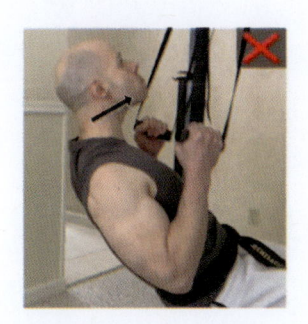

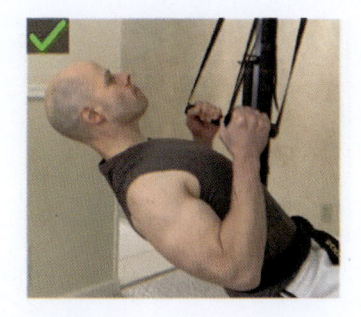

#4 Bring your hands to mid-torso

Some folks like to pull their hands up by their chest while faring their elbows out to the side. Keeping your hands just below your chest or mid-torso will take the stress off your joints while making it easier to keep your arms close to your torso.

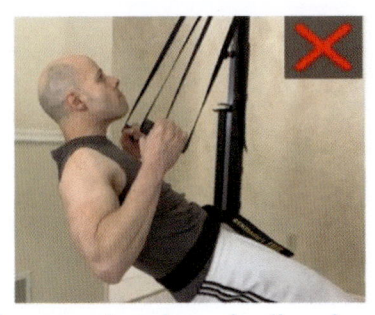

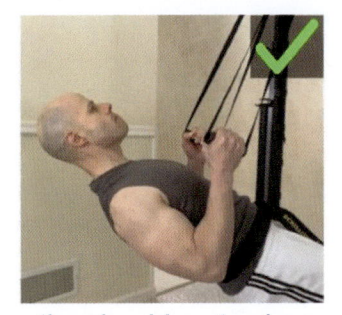

Keeping your hands up by the chest causes the shoulders to shrug and removes tension from the lats. Lowering your hands around mid-torso corrects this.

#5 Maintain a straight wrist

Bending the wrists at the top of a row is another way people try to gain more range of motion without using their back muscles. Curling the wrist at the top of each rep is usually a wasted motion, and it can potentially place some stress on the wrist joint. The solution for this is to keep your wrist straight through each rep.

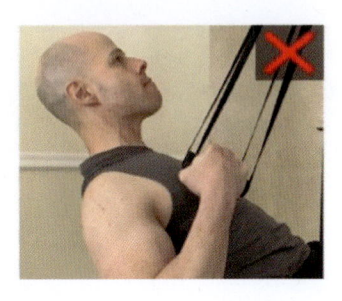

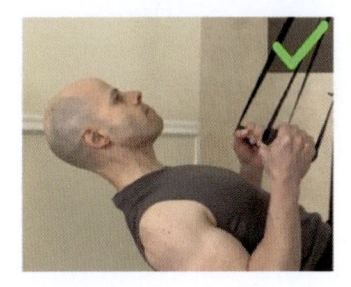

Row progressions

White Belt- Standing Incline Rows

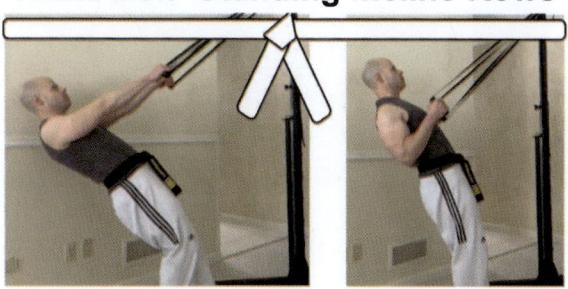

Standing incline rows are a great way to practice your technique, warm up your muscles and lube your stiff joints. They can be incredibly therapeutic if you're sitting all hunched over a desk all day. Practice these with as much range of motion as possible in your arm and shoulder blades. Just like with incline push-ups, you can add resistance by reclining your body back to transfer more of your body weight from your feet to your hands.

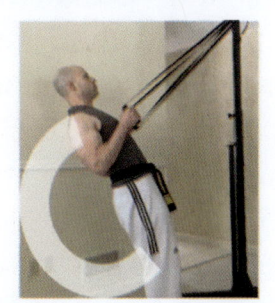

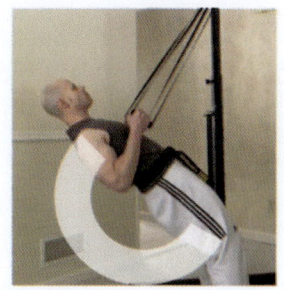

Moving your feet forward places more resistance on your arms.

Yellow Belt- Table Rows

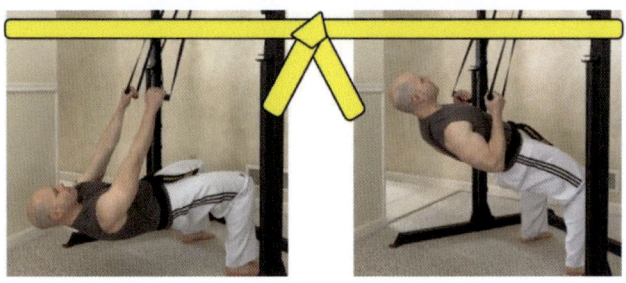

Table rows are the first step that pulls your torso directly against the force of gravity. This angle brings a lot of resistance to your arms and back while requiring more posterior chain stability. Be sure to maintain a steady breathing rhythm and maintain a straight line between your shoulders and knees by keeping your hips extended.

It's easier to set up your table rows from sitting on the floor instead of walking down from a standing position. Just sit on the floor, tense your arms and back, and lift your hips with your hamstrings and glutes. Maintain that position throughout the set and set your hips down on the floor when done. Starting each set this way will improve your posterior chain's tension while making it easier and safer to get into the bottom position.

Green Belt- Straight Leg Rows

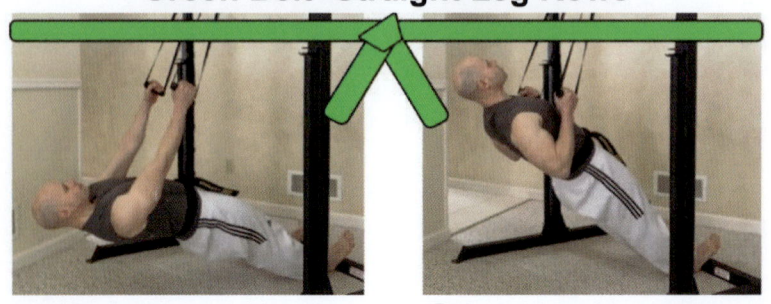

Stretching your legs out straight elongates the lever length of your body. This technique produces more resistance against gravity for both your pulling muscles and supportive posterior chain. Pay close attention to any strain in your lower back. It's imperative to keep your hamstrings and glutes tense so they can handle most of the resistance instead of your lower back.

Just like with the table bridges, it's easier to start this and further progressions from the floor so you can adequately set your posterior tension and body position.

Blue Belt- Elevated Feet Rows

Elevating your feet shifts more of your body weight to your arms, placing more resistance on your pulling muscles. Be aware that a little elevation goes a long way. You probably don't need to elevate your feet more than about a foot or so at first. Also, be sure you're placing your feet on something sturdy, so it doesn't slide or tip, causing your heels to fall and strike the ground. A sturdy chair or weight bench is ideal, or you can have a partner hold your feet up for you.

Red Belt- Single Arm Table Rows

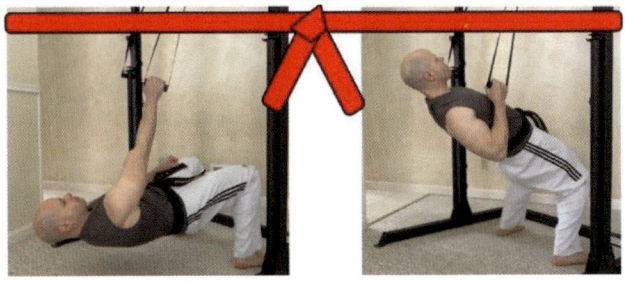

Single-arm rows require a lot of full-body stability and much more pulling strength in the working arm. The key is to pull your working arm into your side as close as possible to minimize the amount of torque on your torso. I recommend using a wide stance when practicing this exercise. You can progress with a more narrow stance as you improve your stability. A slight rotation of the torso is also acceptable.

Black Belt- Straight Leg Single Arm Rows

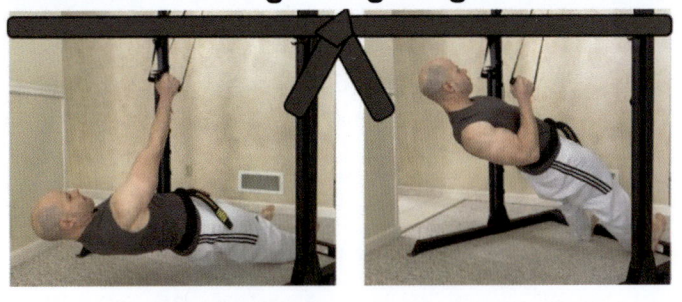

These rows are a lot harder than they look! Once again, they require a ton of upper body strength and full-body stability. Just as with the single-arm table rows, you'll probably want to start with a wide stance and work toward a more narrow foot position over time. Keep in mind that it's natural for the force for the movement to be transferred diagonally through your body. So if you're pulling with your right arm, you'll feel your left leg working harder to maintain stability.

Isometric rows

Isometric rows are a real back-burner, and they do wonders for your tension control and arm strength. Like with push-ups, most folks will only transition through each rep's most challenging point for a fraction of a second. The objective of isometric rows is to find the highest resistance point and then hold that position for time.

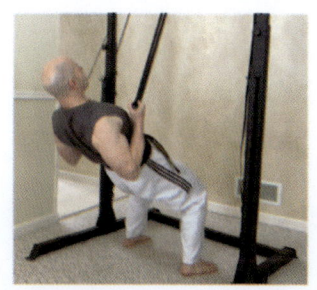

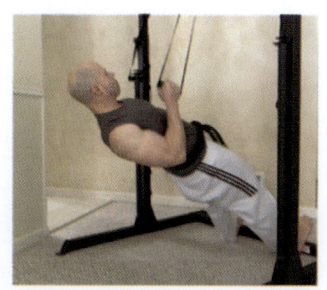

Hold your isometric rows at the top position, where there's more resistance.

Use whatever progression you feel is suitable for you and your strength level. You'll probably find you'll need a more difficult technique for isometrics than you would use for doing reps. These are supposed to be challenging, but you should be able to hold the top position for at least 10 seconds without struggling.

Some people prefer to walk into an isometric row as a way to ease into the exercise. Start in a standing position with your arms flexed as they would be at the top of a row. From there, walk forward while maintaining a flexed arm position until you've applied the amount of resistance you want. This isometric variation can also be done with a single-arm row but be careful of how your weight shifts as you walk forward. Small steps are the key to safely dialing in the perfect level of resistance.

Isometric rows are also an excellent opportunity to learn how to tense up your back muscles and squeeze your arms in toward your centerline. To focus on this, don't just think about holding the top position of the row. Instead, get into the top position and squeeze your arms and shoulder blades inward as much as you can. This slight motion will go a long way in improving your total body stability and joint strength.

Shifting rows

Shifting rows are a unique challenge to test your shoulder and torso stability. They will also apply resistance to your body at angles you'll rarely find on a weight machine or even free weights. This practice not only carries over to very functional arm strength but also bulletproof shoulders and wrists.

Twisting torso rows

Perform these while maintaining the top of the rowing position and slightly twist your torso between your hands. Pay close attention to how you can use the movement in your shoulder blades to create more range of motion in addition to the little action in your arms.

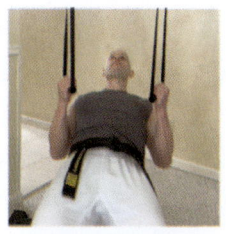

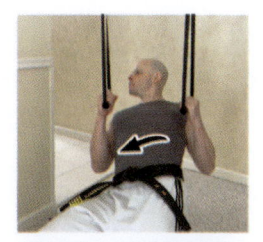

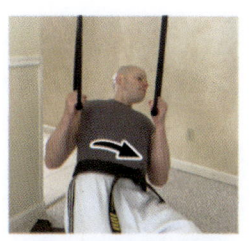

Neutral   **Twist Right**   **Twist Left**

Up and down shifting rows

These shifting rows are not a very large movement, but the devil is in the details. Specifically, these movements integrate not only your arm movement but also your shoulder blades as well. I recommend starting with a moderate level of resistance to get a feel for the move first. You can progress to higher levels of resistance once your shoulders feel more comfortable with the motion.

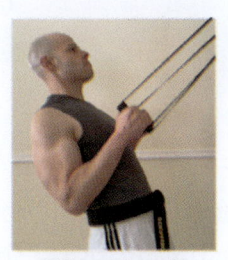

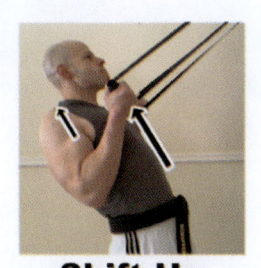

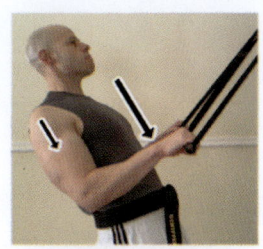

Neutral   **Shift Up**   **Shift Down**

Shifting rows move both of your shoulder blades and hands up and down in a smooth motion.

Archer shifting rows

There are two variations to this exercise, depending on what sort of equipment you may be using. The first variation is similar to the shifting push-ups, where you use a wide hand position and shift your torso from one hand to the other. It's best to practice this exercise on stationary bars or handles.

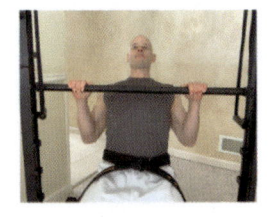

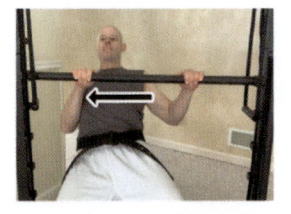

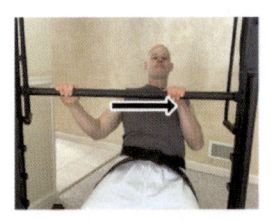

Neutral **Shift Right** **Shift Left**

The second variation is one you'll practice on a mobile setup like a suspension trainer or gymnastics rings. In this case, you keep your torso stationary and move your hands from side to side.

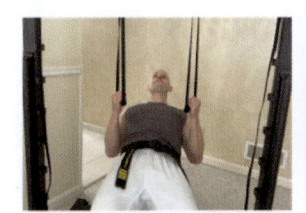

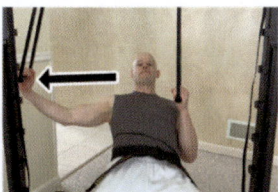

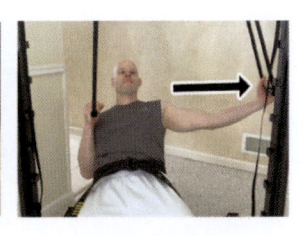

Neutral **Shift Right** **Shift Left**

As with the shifting push-ups, keep most of your weight on the arm that's closer to your torso, and this exercise becomes more difficult the more you reach your arm out to the side.

Circular shifting rows

Circular shifting rows use either stationary or unstable equipment, like suspension straps. Start at the top position, shift to one arm and lower yourself down halfway. Keep your arms bent about 90 degrees. Shift your torso back over to the other arm and pull yourself back up to your hands. Shift back over and repeat for another repetition or reverse the motion.

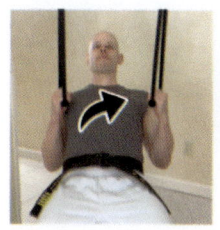

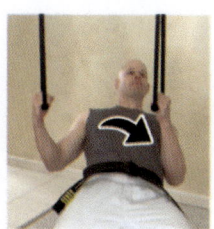

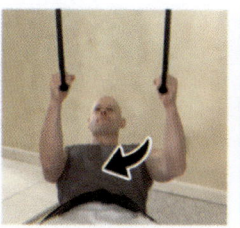

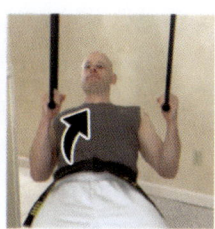

Circular rows are a combination of lateral shifting and rowing movements to work your muscles in various angles.

Explosive rows

Explosive rows are a bit tricky to execute due to the risk of injury from falling from whatever you're grabbing. I recommend using a bit more resistance than you would for explosive push-ups, so you're not creating a lot of momentum that's throwing you off your support. If you're using rings or suspension trainers, use enough resistance so you're not floating at the top and creating slack in the straps. This slack can create a jerking shock when your bodyweight lands back into the handle. This jerking motion can wear out the suspension trainer and compromise your secure support. It can also be stressful on your joints.

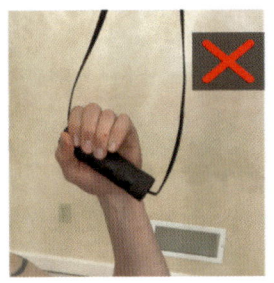

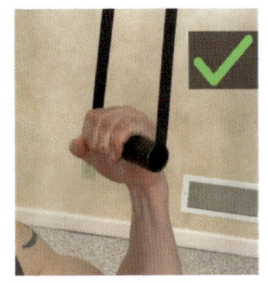

Row hard and fast; just try not to create a lot of momentum and slack to make a high-impact catch.

Accelerated rows

Perform these with a fast concentric motion, sort of like you're trying to elbow someone behind you as hard as you can. At the top, hold for half a second and lower yourself under control. Pause again at the bottom to kill any momentum and then pull yourself up again with accelerated force

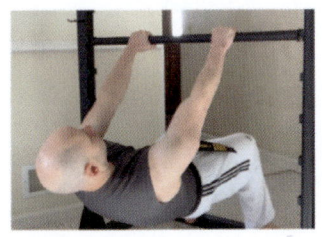

Pause at Bottom **Pull Up Fast** **Pause at Top**

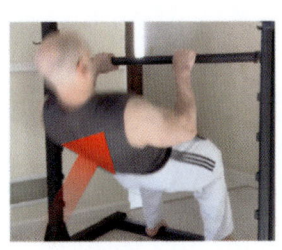

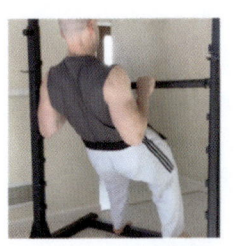

Pump rows

These are just like the pump push-ups but in reverse. Pull yourself up hard as if you're trying to hit your chest against your hands and immediately lower your torso down to the floor in a quick, controlled motion. At the bottom, quickly reverse direction and pull yourself back up. Complete the number of reps in a smooth action without any sudden jerks or stops. If you're doing this on a suspension trainer, you can smooth out the motion with a slight circular movement of your hands, sort of like you're using a rowing machine.

Keep in mind that you can progress the resistance of these two moves to make them more challenging. I much prefer to use more resistance and maintain contact with whatever I'm grabbing for safety reasons than to pull hard enough to either hit the underside of a bar or jerk hard on a set of suspension straps.

Chapter 5

Building Rock-Solid Legs

In the world of strength, squats reign supreme, but lunges are king when it comes to martial arts. That's because you're not just using this unsung hero of leg training to build raw leg strength, heck no! As a martial artist, you know brute force just won't cut it. You need mobility, unshakable stability, and explosive power that rivals a lightning bolt. That's the real reason for practicing lunges. They will help you build a complete lower body conditioning program, one that leaves no stone unturned, so you don't get caught flat-footed in the ring or life.

Key technical points

#1 Focus on bringing your hips closer to your front heel

Lunges are unilateral squat movements. They are essentially a single-leg squat with rear leg stability and support.

Squats can be extremely technical, but I prefer to keep things simple. Instead of thinking about every joint and muscle in your lower body, focus on bringing your hips closer to the back of your front heel. This motion will ensure a proper technique for every rep with clockwork consistency.

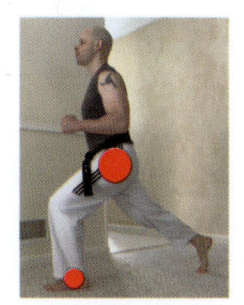

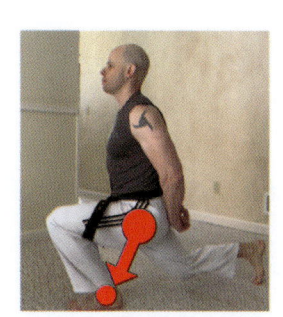

Focus on pulling your hip closer to the back of your front heel

#2 Place your front foot near your centerline and track the knee in slightly

Lunges mimic the natural motion of walking where you place one foot in front of the other. As bipedal humans, we evolved to move with our feet moving underneath us, which means keeping your feet close to your centerline. Doing this requires a slight inward angle of your thigh.

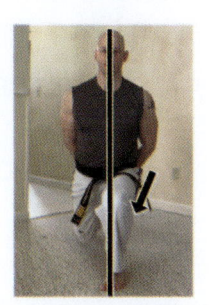

Keep your hips level as your knee points slightly to your centerline to avoid stress on the joints.

This slight inward angle also does a lot for your hip strength and mobility, which is also crucial in martial arts training.

Also, be sure your toes point forward and not out to the side, which can create excessive torque on the knee joint.

#3 Keep your back foot vertical except during instep lunges

Lunges primarily work your front leg, but your back leg still receives some strength and stability conditioning. It's not uncommon for some people to struggle to control their back foot, and it tends to twist to the side.

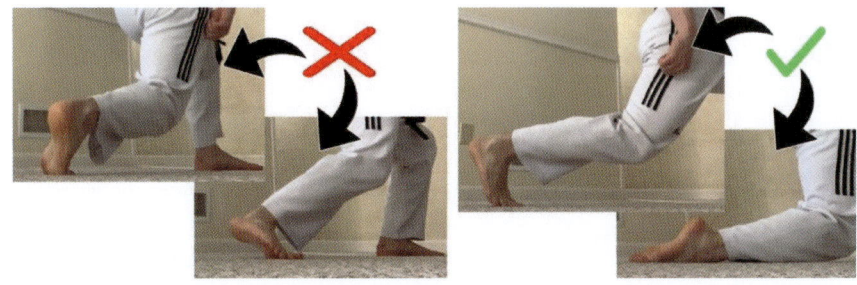

Avoid letting your foot twist to the inside or outside during lunges.

This instability is usually a case of weak hips with trouble keeping the whole leg stable at the bottom of the lunge position. If your back foot is twisting or tilting, regress the exercise a level or two until your hip stability improves.

#4 Maintain an upright torso

Lunges are a total body exercise, especially when it comes to stability and control. All of the leg strength in the world won't help you if your core is weak and unstable. Maintaining an upright torso during lunges improves your core control and integrates your upper body stability with your lower body strength.

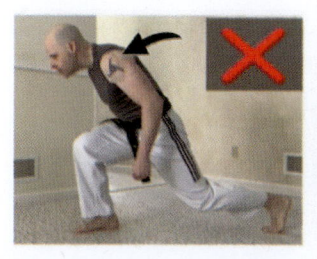

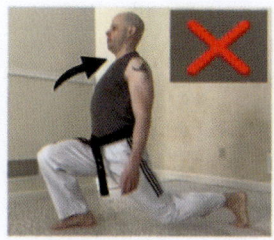

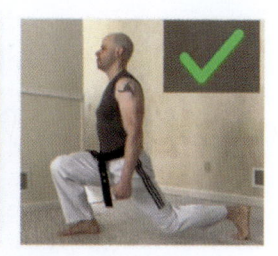

#5 Press into the floor with your front heel

"Dancing heels" are one of the most common issues athletes face while practicing lunges. Excessive foot movement happens when there's a lack of tension along the back of the leg and your weight shifts onto the ball of the front foot. The result is there's almost no weight on your heel, which compromises your stability while also placing a lot of stress on your knee. The sweet spot for weight distribution is the front of the heel or on the arch's backside in your foot.

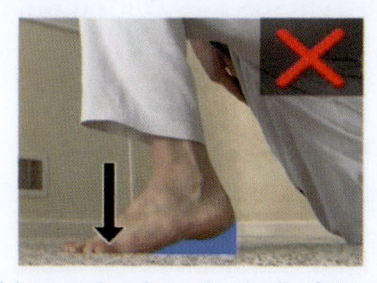

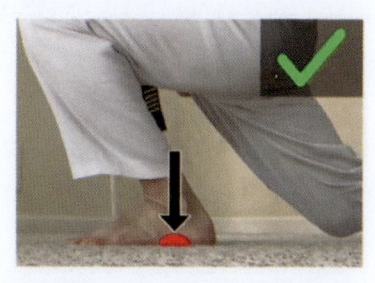

Avoid pressing into the ball of the foot and lifting the heel. Maintain tension in the hamstrings to press the heel into the floor to keep a flat foot.

Lunge progressions

White Belt- Standing Knee Tuck

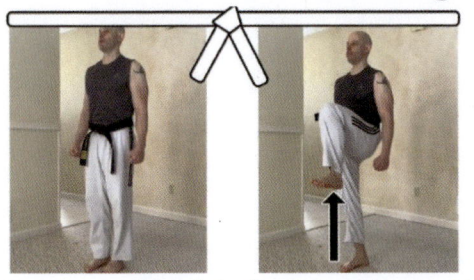

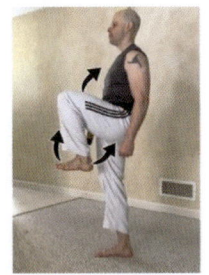

Focus on the triple flexion of the ankle, knee, and hip joints.

As Han Solo once said; "She may not look like much, but she's got it where it counts kid," and that's certainly the case with standing knee tucks. Sure, this doesn't look like a typical lunge, but it still completes the hip-to-heel movement pattern. These are the opposite motion of lunges as you keep your body in place and move your leg instead of the other way around. Nonetheless, this motion is critical for learning how to pull your heel and hip together which is the key to optimal lunge training.

This pulling motion is the secret to practicing lunges with more stability, strength, and mobility. It also eliminates stress on the front of the knee while creating balanced muscle tension throughout the leg. Naturally, training to pick your knee up is the key to improving your kicks as well.

Yellow Belt- Stationary Lunges

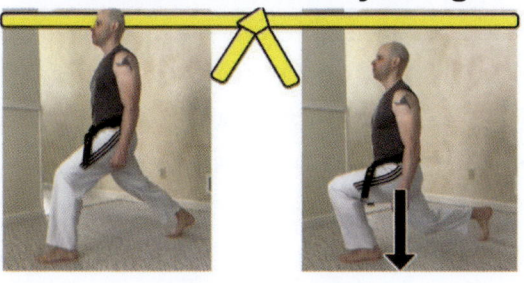

Stationary lunges are sometimes referred to as split squats since they closely resemble a squatting motion. Stand in a staggered stance and "squat" down on your front leg while your back leg provides support. This exercise teaches you how to transfer the pulling action from the standing knee tuck to a traditional lunge motion.

Start off keeping a 50/50 weight distribution between your two legs and progress by shifting more weight to your front leg as you feel ready. Try to work up to having 70-80% of your weight on the front leg at the bottom of each rep.

Green Belt- Spot Lunge

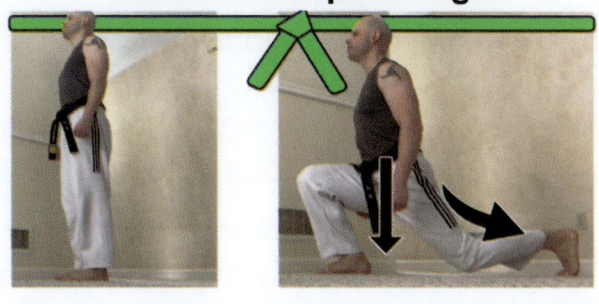

Spot lunges are the next level since they require more coordination and stability as you alternate between your two legs. I always recommend doing back spot lunges where you step back with your supporting leg and drop your body weight down on your front foot. This variation helps you maintain optimal weight placement on your front leg and prevents a dancing heel. It also helps you learn how to pull yourself forward with your glutes and hamstrings when you stand up just as you would while walking or running.

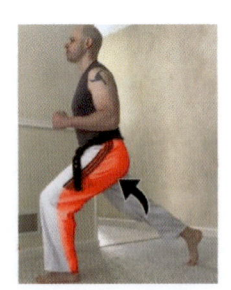

Using the glutes and hamstrings of the front leg to pull your hips up and forward rather than pushing off the floor with the back leg.

Blue Belt- Walking Lunges

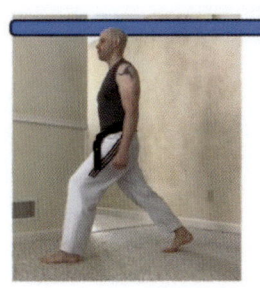

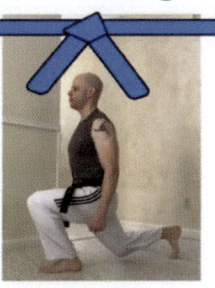

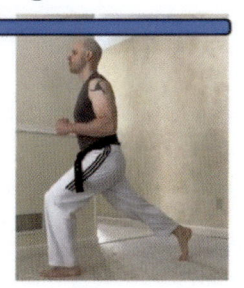

Walking lunges teach you how to step and decelerate your body in a safe and controlled manner. It's easy to fall slightly forward when stepping which compromises your power and control. It also creates a lot of stress on the front of the leg putting a strain on the knee and shin.

The resulting knee stress is why you want to step-and-sink into each lunge and then pull-and-lift out of each step for balanced and complete lower body development.

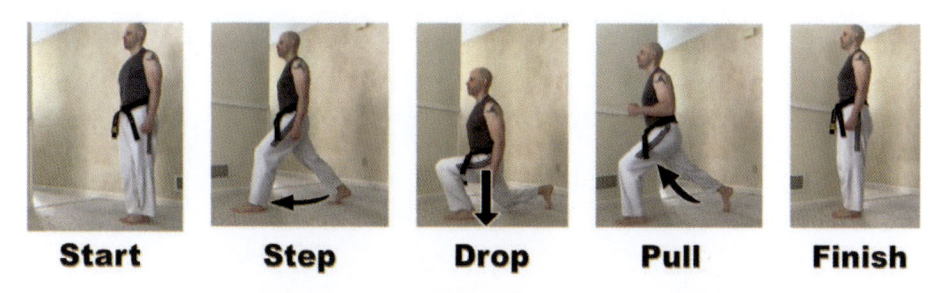

Start   **Step**   **Drop**   **Pull**   **Finish**

Red Belt- Walking Twist Lunges

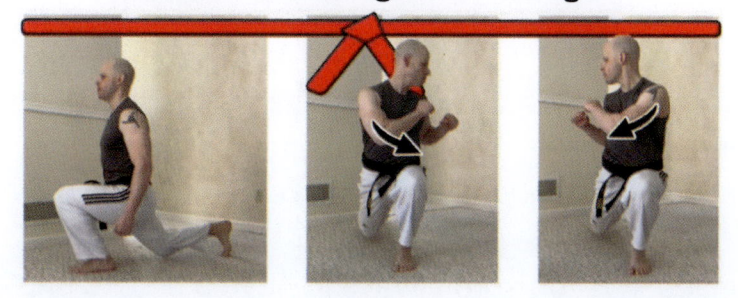

These are a bit of a shifting exercise as your torso's twisting action requires the muscles in your lower body to be stable in a variety of positions. This exercise also makes your legs work harder as an isometric while you twist side to side.

You can progress this technique with three basic variations. The first step is to practice twisting side to side while holding the bottom position. The next level of difficulty is to twist at the bottom of spot lunges, where you step back and twist. The most challenging variation is to rotate in both directions at the bottom of each step during walking lunges.

It's natural to feel stronger when you twist toward your back leg and less stable twisting to your front leg. If twisting toward the front leg is too tricky, rotate to the hind leg on each lunge for now and add the other side after a few weeks.

Black Belt- Overhead Lunges

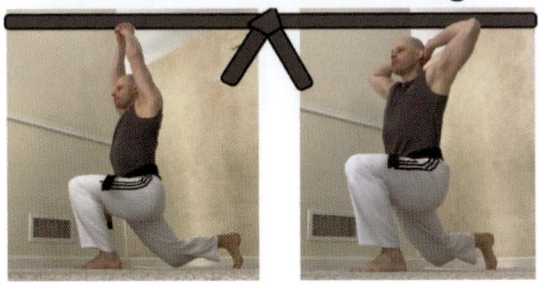

Overhead lunges create a top-heavy movement when your arms are reaching overhead. This effect is amplified even more if you're holding onto weight like a dumbbell or even a heavy book. Rocks are also a useful tool for adding weight to your lunges. Just be sure always to have a secure grip on whatever you're holding, so you don't accidentally drop it on yourself.

Being top-heavy requires much more strength and stability from your lower body, plus you improve the balance and mobility of your upper body at the same time.

If reaching overhead is a bit much, you can use a "prisoner lunge" when you place your hands on your head's back. Prisoner lunges will still make you top-heavy while giving you a point of contact with your hands. It's also an excellent way to work your upper back as you pull your elbows back instead of letting them move slightly inward.

Isometric lunges

Isometric lunges are a fantastic way to make your legs stronger and more resilient. They will quickly improve your stability and weight distribution while also loosening up your hips and ankle joints. They are also handy for building up your leg strength if you're a beginner or coming back from an injury.

I highly recommend practicing your isometric lunges from the ground up. Starting at the bottom helps ensure proper body position and weight distribution without feeling too unsteady while getting into position.

Begin with your back knee on the ground and both knees at about a 90-degree angle. You may want to put a folded towel or pad under your back knee for comfort. Shift as much weight as you can onto your front leg while maintaining pressure on your front heel. From there, press down into your front foot and lift your back knee about an inch off the floor. Hold that position for time and gently bring your knee back down before switching to do the same on the other leg.

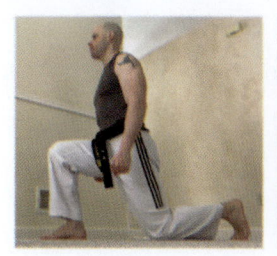

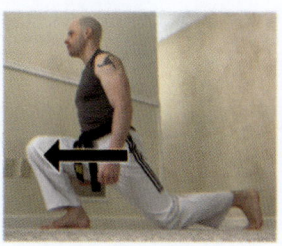

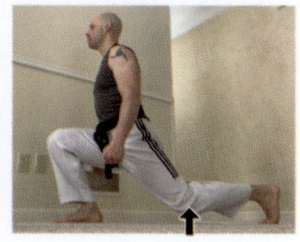

You may wish to hold onto something sturdy if you find it difficult to remain stable for more than a few seconds. You can progress by gradually removing your upper body support over time.

If holding the bottom isometric position is too difficult, you can start with an isometric split squat. Start in a staggered stance and squat down as low as you feel you can and hold. Be sure to hold onto something with your upper body to help pull yourself out of the bottom position as your front leg may become too fatigued to push yourself back up. Start from the floor once you can maintain a deep lunge comfortably.

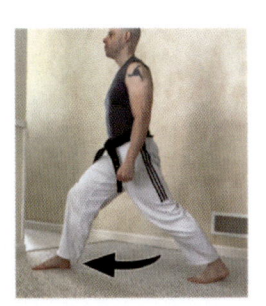

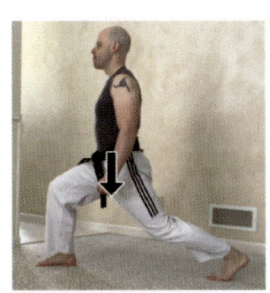

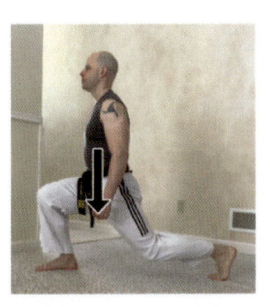

You can start isometric lunges from a standing position by stepping forward and then dropping your weight straight down.

Shifting lunges

Shifting lunges are some of the best exercises for building a strong lower body foundation. They shore up any weaknesses in your strength, mobility, and stability, helping you become strong in various positions.

Front and back shifting lunges

The first variation works the shifting strength along your sagittal plane. Squat down into a low isometric lunge and shift your weight front and back between your two feet. Be sure to keep your torso upright, so the motion comes from moving your hips rather than your upper body.

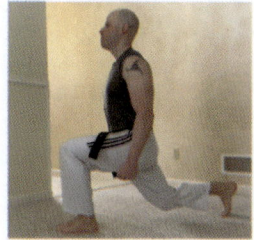

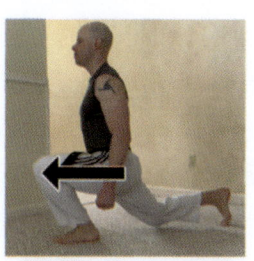

Start Neutral **Shift Forward** **Shift Back**

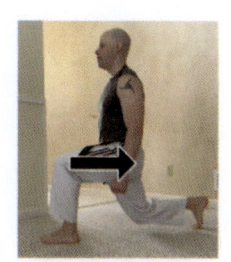

Try your best to keep the heel of your front foot on the floor although you may slightly shift your weight to the ball of your foot. And yes, it's perfectly safe to move your knee over your toes. Stress on the knee is from a lack of tension along the back of your leg.

Side to side shifting lunges

Lunges have limited lateral shifting motion, but there is some movement you can work on. As with front and back shifting lunges, focus on moving your hips laterally instead of your torso. Just be sure to move in a smooth and controlled motion at all times.

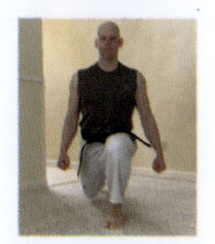

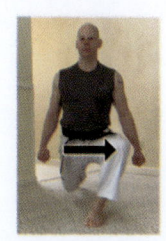

Start Neutral **Shift Outward** **Shift Inward**

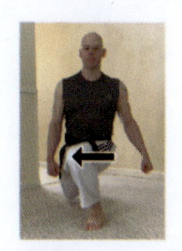

Explosive lunges

Fast legs create fast athletes. Powerful legs not only help you run and jump but also kick and dodge out of the way. Unfortunately, explosive unilateral leg training can be a bit riskier if you haven't developed enough strength and stability. These explosive lunge progressions will give you the options you need to build power at any level of ability.

Accelerated split squats

These are an excellent place to start to develop the feeling of driving your front foot straight down into the floor. Bring yourself down into a low lunge position, pause at the bottom and then forcefully drive your foot into the floor to push yourself upward. Pause at the top and repeat. Remember, you can progress this exercise by how low you squat down and regress it by using a more shallow range of motion.

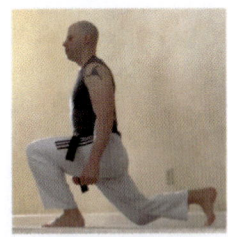

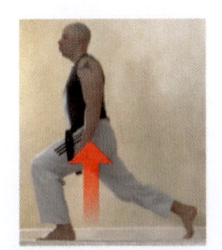

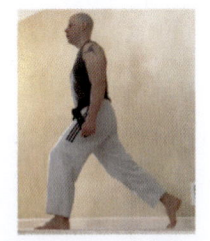

Start Low   **Push Up Fast**   **Pause at Top**

Pump split squats

These help you learn the coordination and stability you need to use your legs in a smooth, yet powerful way. You'll use the same split squat technique as before where you'll be squatting down on your front leg, but now you'll eliminate the pause at the top and bottom of each rep. Try your best to prevent a sudden or jerky motion and aim for a smooth transition at the top and bottom of each rep.

Skipping

The rest of the explosive lunges require a jumping motion where you'll need to power off the balls of your feet. Skipping is a fun and natural way to develop this sort of power without asking too much from the bigger muscles in your legs. You can also do this while driving one knee up to develop your hips in a similar way to kicking.

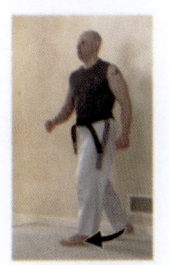

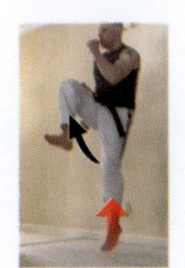

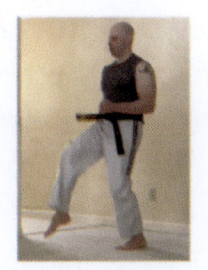

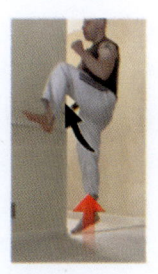

Skipping should be done in a smooth motion by stepping forward and then jumping off the front foot while driving up with the back knee. Land gently on the jumping foot and repeat by driving up with the other knee.

Switchfoot lunges

Explosive lunges often require shifting your legs back and forth. This movement can be a little tricky to learn if you haven't done it before.

That's why I recommend practicing a switchfoot technique where you jump only an inch or two off the floor and quickly switch feet. The longer and deeper your stance is, the more difficult this exercise becomes. When warming up, start with a short stance and work your way to a longer one as you feel comfortable.

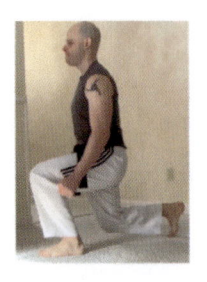

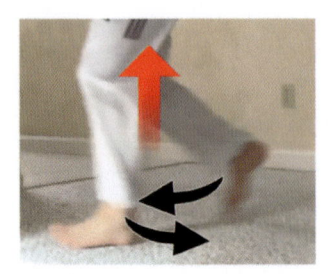

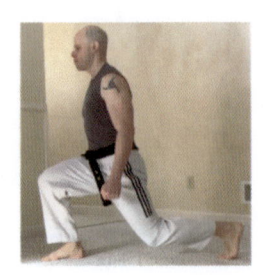

Jump lunges

Lastly, we have the ultimate explosive lunge where you power off your front leg, switch in mid-air, and land back in the opposite stance. These are essentially assisted single-leg jumping squats as you primarily push off your front leg. These are done just like the switchfoot lunges, only now you're trying to jump as high as you can when you switch feet. Be aware of your weight shifting onto your back leg while doing these. This shift isn't a bad thing, but it does remove weight from your front leg and can put more stress on your back knee.

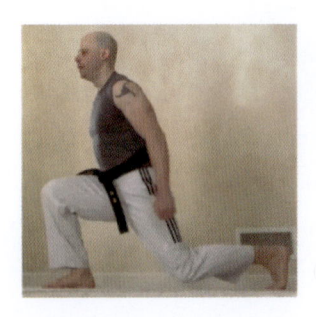

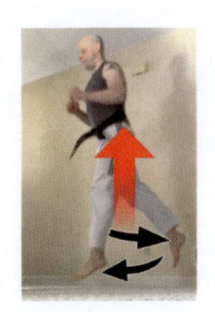

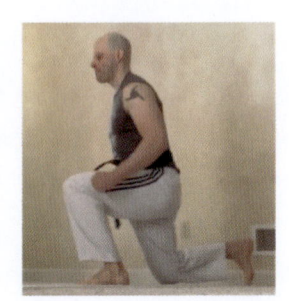

Chapter 6

Build Punch-Proof Abs With Leg Raises

There are many abdominal exercises out there, but when it comes to martial arts training, nothing comes close to leg raises.

The reason for the leg raise superiority is simple; many forms of human movement require picking up and controlling your legs in space. Even the simple activity of walking requires you to pick your foot off the ground.

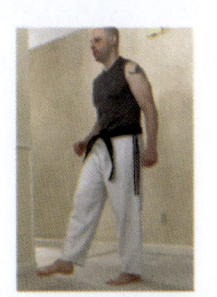

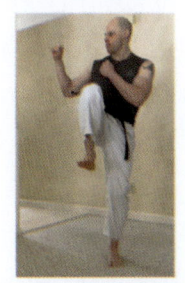

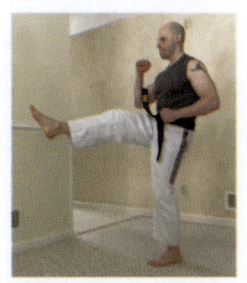

Most lower body movement requires a stable core and mobile hips whether you're kicking or simply stepping forward.

Of course, we martial artists are in a performance league all our own. You need to pick your legs up for kicks and even some stances. Strong abdominals and hips are also important for groundwork and wrestling. A stronger set of abdominals can also help you fend off blows to the gut. The bottom line is you need a strong ability to flex your hips and abdominals for both offense and defense. I pity those who neglect this form of training.

Key technical points

#1 Maintain tension along the front of your legs

You'll gain the most benefit, with less stress on your back, if you keep the entire front side of your body tense. Focus on tensing your hips, quads, and even your shins. Pulling your toes up helps maintain this sort of tension.

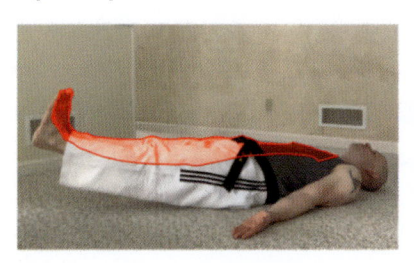

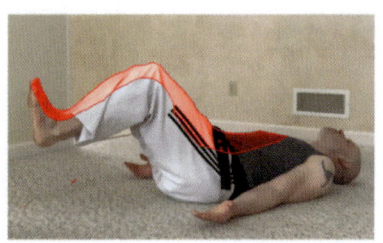

Maintaining a little tension along the front of your body is key with both bent and straight leg variations.

#2 Keep your abs tense through the full range of motion

One of the most common mistakes is letting the abdominals relax as you lower your feet to the floor. It's an easy thing to do since it's more challenging to keep a muscle tense as it stretches out. It's especially common since even many athletes have poor tension control in their abs.

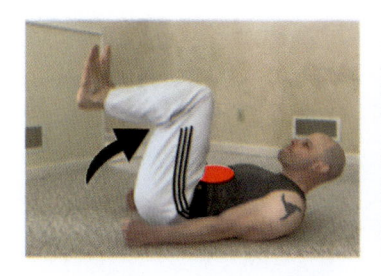

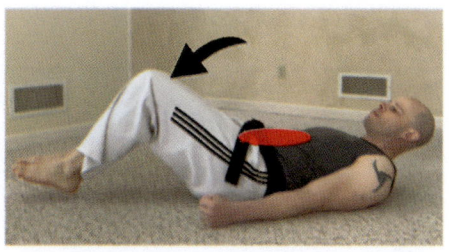

Maintaining tension at the bottom of each rep will support your lumbar spine.

The result is a lot of abdominal tension is produced at the very top of each rep when your abs contract and they relax as soon as you start lowering your legs. To prevent your abdominals from resting, practice keeping your abs as tense as possible through the full range of motion. You may need to regress the exercise several steps to practice this effectively, but don't worry, maintaining tension through the full range of motion will make your core training much more effective.

#3 Focus on pulling up your pelvis

Your abdominal muscles don't lift your legs. They aren't even attached to your legs at all. Instead, they connect to your pubic bone at the base of your pelvis. So the real purpose of leg raises is to move and control your pelvis as you use your hips to lift your legs. It also makes your core more stable giving you total body control and agility while kicking and changing stances.

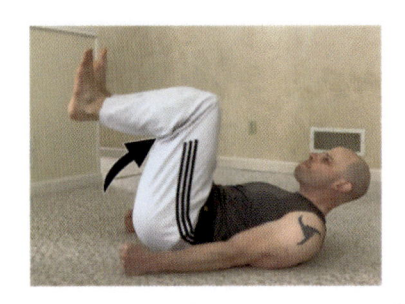

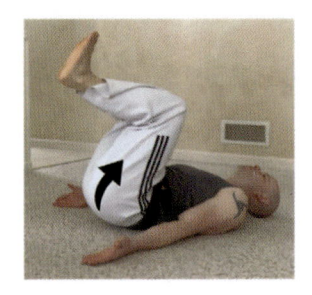

The photo on the left shows how I lift my legs but my hips stay on the floor. On the right, I'm lifting my hips up to fully contract my abdominals.

#4 Keep feet together

You may discover a slight strength imbalance between your right and left leg which can cause one leg to lift faster than the other. Keeping your feet together while lifting your legs will iron out any such imbalances.

#5 Keep your shoulders packed

Leg raises work the front of your body which means you'll need to maintain stability in your back. Packing your shoulders down and back, even when lying on the floor, will create all the posterior stability you need so your abdominals can work as effectively as possible.

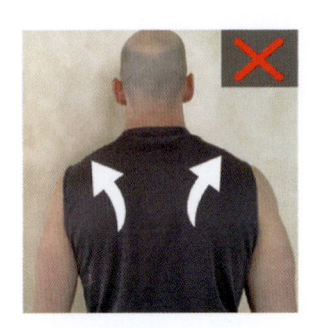

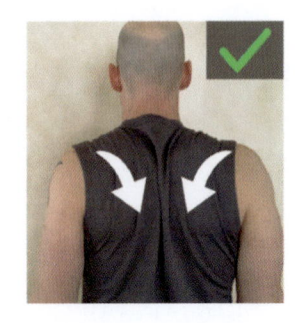

Leg raise progressions

White Belt- Hollow Body Hold

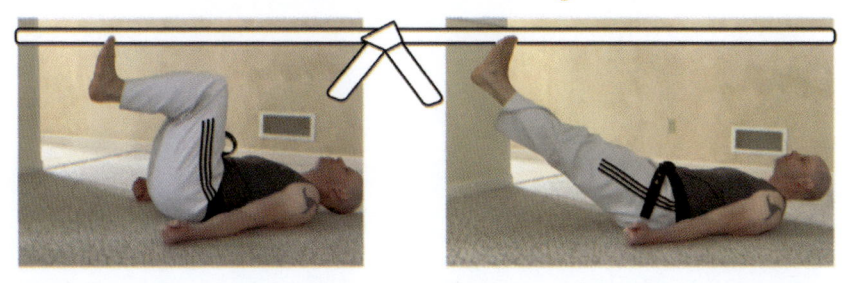

Holding your legs out straight, or bent in as an isometric exercise is a great way to strengthen your abs while improving tension control and breathing.

The hollow body hold is an ideal exercise for learning how to maintain tension along the front of your body in an isometric position. Start in a tucked position and slowly extend your legs outward. Maintain tension in your abs while keeping your lower back on the floor. The lower your feet are the more difficult it will be to maintain abdominal tension. Hold for time and finish each set by gently lowering your feet to the floor.

Yellow Belt- Knee Tucks

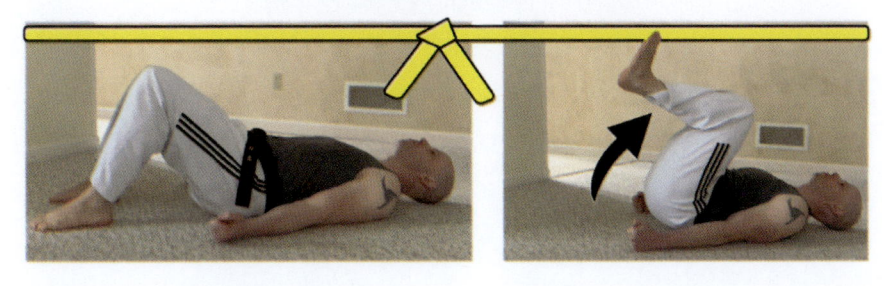

Knee tucks help you practice flexing your hips and crunching your abs through a short range of motion. This technique will help you learn how to keep your abs tense and stable as you move your legs at the hip joint. Be sure to lift your legs in a smooth motion without a lot of momentum so you can raise your hips off the floor with the strength of your abdominals.

Green Belt- Straight Leg Raises

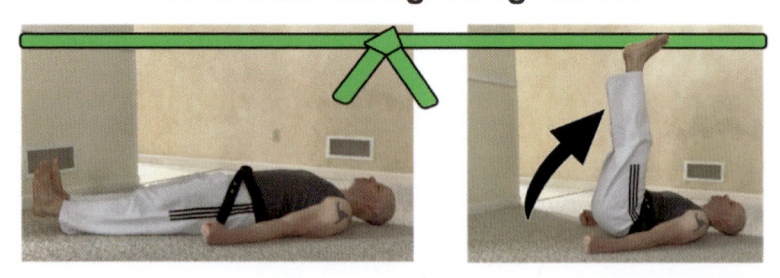

Straight leg raises progress the bent knee raise several ways. They require a more extensive range of motion as your hips extend further to lower your knees close to the floor. Second, your extended legs place more resistance on your hips which also requires more strength in your abs to stabilize your pelvis. These can also help you learn how to breathe while keeping your abs tense which is vital for endurance during sparring.

Blue Belt- Hanging Knee Raises

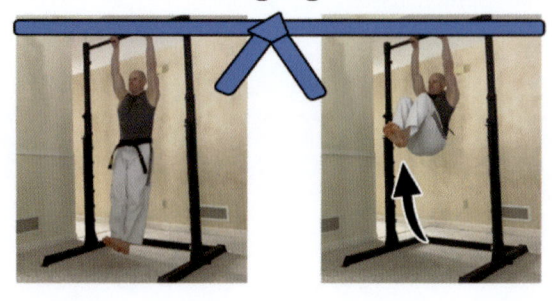

Once again, this progression steps up the challenge a couple of ways. Hanging requires a lot more strength and stability in your shoulders and back. You'll also need a lot more hip and abdominal strength to lift your legs directly against the pull of gravity. Lastly, you no longer have a solid floor to support your lower back and hips so your lats and traps will have to stay tense to provide support. On the plus side, no longer having your hips against the floor gives you more freedom to lift or tuck up your pelvis.

I recommend keeping your feet slightly forward at the bottom position and lifting them as straight up as possible. This keeps most of your momentum in check and helps prevent swinging since you're moving in a vertical motion.

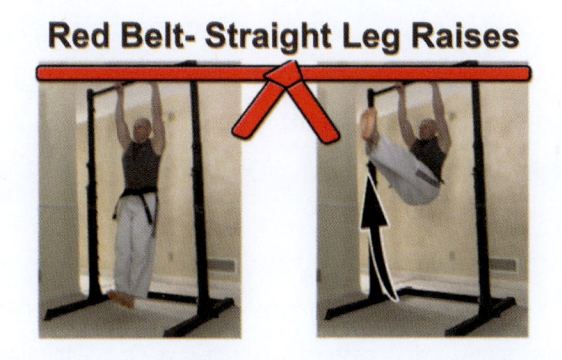

Red Belt- Straight Leg Raises

Just as on the floor, straightening out your legs will increase the resistance on your hips and require more stability from your abdominals. If straight legs are too challenging, bend your knees halfway, note that straight leg raises can create a lot more momentum and potential swinging from your body. You can prevent swinging with more tension in your back and keeping your feet in front of you at the bottom of each rep.

Black Belt- Straight Leg Raises With a Pause

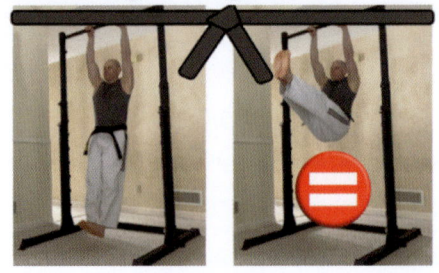

Leg raises are almost always done with some degree of momentum especially when hanging from an overhead support. Having a little momentum isn't bad, but it does make the exercise significantly easier. That's why the ultimate level in this program is to lift your legs and hold the top position for 2-3 seconds. Expect your legs to dip down a few inches the first time you do this due to how difficult it is to hold that top position for even a second. You can further progress this exercise by lifting, and holding, your legs at a higher elevation.

Isometric Leg Raises

Isometric leg raises are all about stability and control. They are a great place to start if you haven't been doing core work for a while or need to improve tension control. They are also very challenging for advanced athletes depending on which progression you are using.

The most important consideration is the level of resistance you employ. Use enough resistance to challenge yourself after about 20 or 30 seconds but don't use so much that you can't hold the position for more than a moment or feel a strain in your lower back. Keep in mind that isometric exercises can be performed with slightly more resistance than you would use for dynamic repetition work.

Setting yourself up is pretty simple. You lift your legs and hold. If you are practicing a straight leg variation, I recommend lifting your knees up and then extending your legs out to apply the resistance rather than lifting your legs with momentum and then struggling to hold them up.

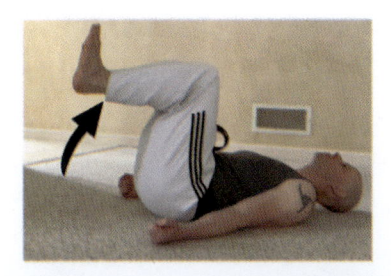

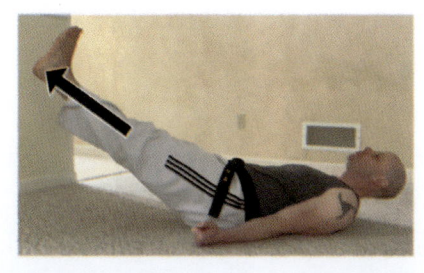

Bend and extend! It's much easier to set up your position and tension control compared to just lifting your legs up straight.

Isometric leg raises are also very good for improving abdominal tension control. A simple trick to improving this is to place a weight or even press down into your abdominals while holding up your legs. Keeping your abs braced to push against your hand, or the weight is a great way to improve the mind-muscle connection in your abdominals.

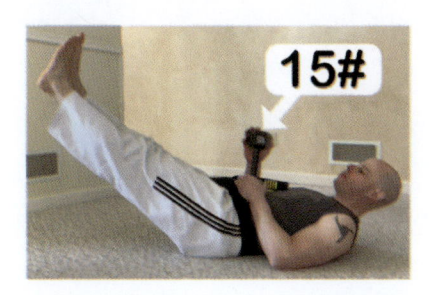

Shifting leg raise

Shifting work is an ideal way to break out of the sagittal plane and incorporate some twisting or side-to-side motion. Shifting leg raises will also help build more stability in your lumbar spine as well as target your obliques.

Side to side leg raise

The first shifting variation is to lift your legs side to side before returning to the center and lowering them back down. If you are doing lying leg raises you may want to place your arms out to the side for stability.

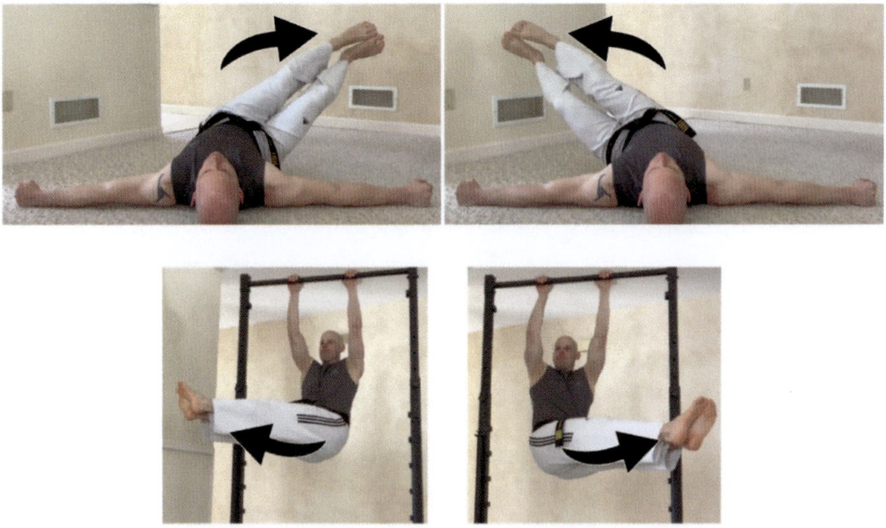

Side-to-side shifting can be done by laying on the floor or hanging.

Alternating leg raise

Alternating leg raises are another variation that builds mobility and control in your hips and core. This variation has an exceptional amount of carryover to kicking strength where one leg remains close to the floor for stability as you lift the other.

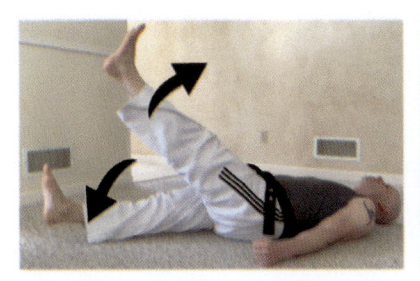

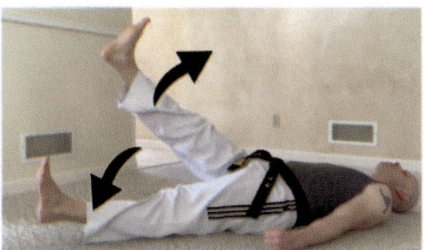

Alternating leg raises involve moving both legs at the same time with one leg lifting and the other lowering.

Feel free to experiment with the various speeds with alternating leg raises, but try to maintain a smooth and controlled motion at all times. Excessive speed can place a lot of stress on the lumbar spine if you're not warmed up.

Circle leg raise

Circling leg raises are the third variation where you move your legs in a circular motion. You can practice these doing all of your reps clockwise and then resting a bit before doing them counterclockwise. You can also alternate your reps which forces you to stop and reverse direction after each rep.

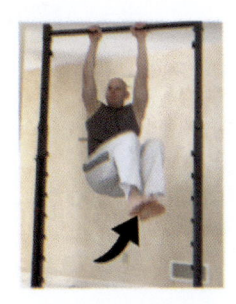

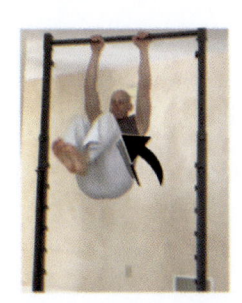

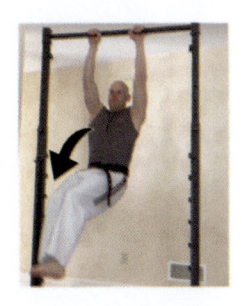

Explosive leg raises

As with your explosive rows, powerful leg raises should emphasize a smooth and controlled motion rather than a lot of fast movement with jerky starts and stops.

A key point with powerful leg raises is to actively pull your legs down rather than letting your core relax so gravity does the work for you. Pulling down will help to emphasize continuous tension on the front side of your body while smoothing out the transition between lifting and lowering your legs with each rep. If you're lying on the floor, you may find it helpful to hang onto something sturdy to give you some support while moving your lower body in a fast motion.

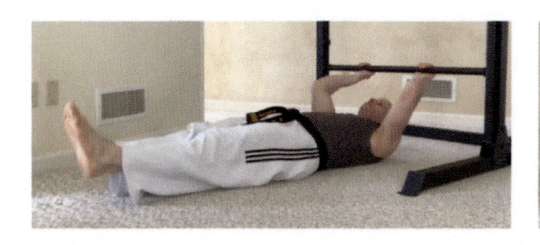

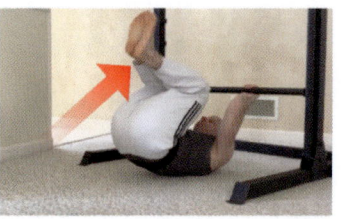

As with all explosive work, it's perfectly acceptable to have some momentum as you lift your legs. Just be sure your abs don't relax as the momentum carries your legs up.
Continuous tension is key.

Chapter 7

Accessory Exercises to Strengthen Weak Links

These accessory moves resemble some classical martial arts techniques you might practice in your forms. They are not necessarily the most practical bread-n-butter movements, but they can do wonders for shoring up weak links. Feel free to consider these optional, but play around with them and see if you can unlock some hidden potential.

Grip work

Years ago, I spent a winter indoor rock climbing, and I was amazed by how much a stronger grip carried over to punching power. I felt like my hands turned into indestructible hammers. Grip strength also does wonders for grabbing and manipulating your opponent.

The simplest and most efficient way to improve your grip strength is to hang from a set of towels during your usual pulling exercises. Using a towel grip during rows or hanging work also works your grip without adding extra activities to your routine.

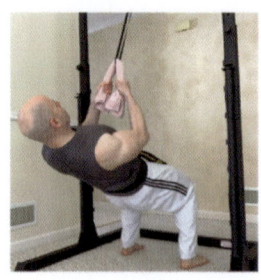

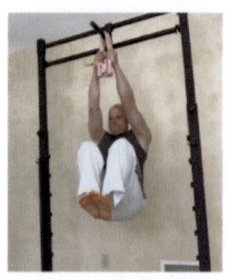

Grabbing a towel during rows and hanging exercises will build a vice-like grip in no time.

You can also practice grip training in its own right by hanging from an overhead bar for time. Using a wrapped towel to make the bar thicker can even make hanging more difficult. Lastly, you can wear thick winter gloves to add thickness to the bar and increase your grip strength.

Neck strengthening

A strong neck is an invaluable defense line, especially in wrestling and striking martial arts, where you may experience blows to the chin.

Understandably, some coaches get nervous when it comes to training in the neck due to supporting your vertebrae, which surround a plethora of sensitive nerves. This observation of physical anatomy is why I strongly recommend using an isometric approach so you avoid any movement that can increase your risk of injury. I also advise practicing on an elevated surface like a weight bench or piece of furniture. This technique positions your torso, so you don't press down into your neck with your bodyweight.

Front Neck Work

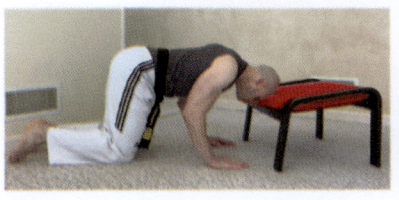

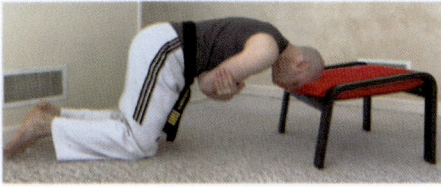

Front neck work is best done on the knees at first, using your hands for support as you get into position. Add resistance by placing less pressure in your hands until you can fold your arms across your chest.

Back Neck Work

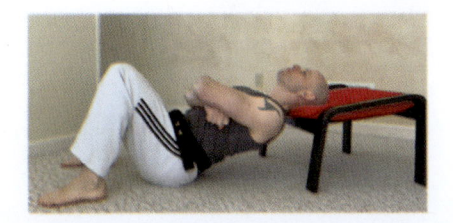

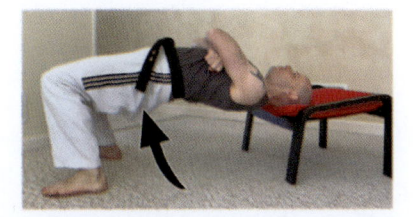

Practice Back neck exercises facing up, starting with your hips on the floor. Lifting your hips places resistance on your entire posterior chain, especially the back of your neck. The higher you raise, the more resistance you'll place on your neck.

These isometric neck drills are easy to adjust the resistance depending on how far you place your feet from your head's contact point. You can also set your hands on the floor with the front neck variation to add additional support. Start with your knees or hips on the floor, respectively, tense your neck muscles and gently lift your hips to apply resistance. Note that the higher you lift, the more resistance you'll place on your neck, so don't feel you need to raise very high at first. Use a conservative approach while you build up the strength and confidence in your neck muscles.

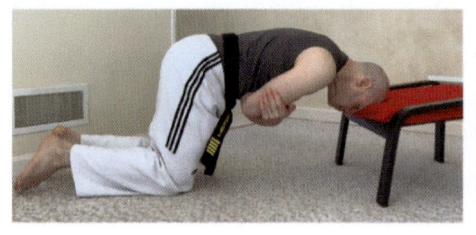

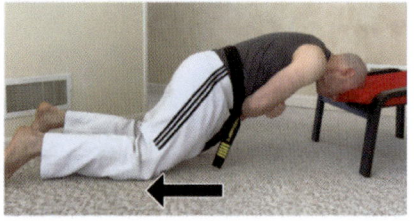

Extending your body adds resistance to the exercise. Start with your hips bent at a 90-degree angle and work up to a straight torso. Eventually, you may get strong enough to do this with your whole body in a straight line between your head and feet.

Hip work

Your hips are some of the most critical muscles for total body control, but unfortunately, weak hips are common for modern-day martial artists. Naturally, the strength and stability of your hips also dramatically affect your kicking proficiency.

The simplest way to strengthen and improve your hips' mobility is to lift a straight leg out in front of you and hold that position. Be sure to treat this as a strengthening exercise rather than a dynamic kick or stretch. Lock both legs by putting tension in every muscle in your lower body. Lift one leg while keeping the other straight and pause at the top for a good five or ten seconds before returning the leg down under control. Repeat for reps or alternate to the other leg.

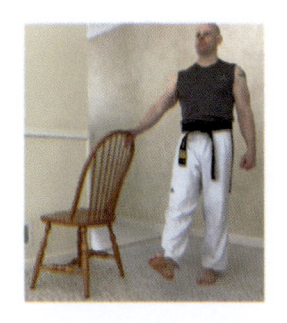

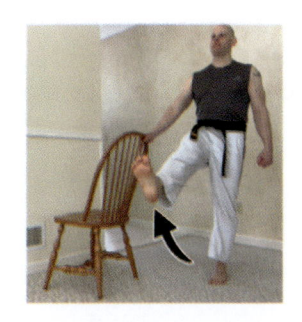

The other variation is to lift the leg to your back or side. Again, use this as a strengthening exercise to lift your leg with minimum momentum and hold the top position for five to ten seconds. Unlike with the front leg raise, the side leg raise uses a tilted torso.

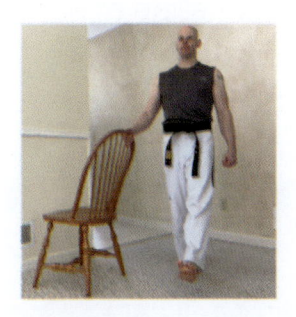

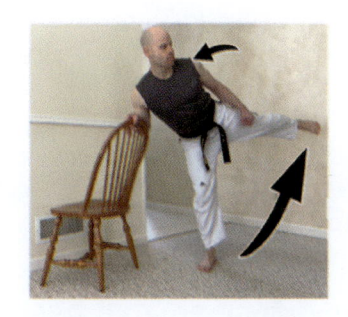

A fun variation is to swing the leg from the front raise position to the back position and return it to the front, sort of like a high sweeping kick with a straight leg. This movement will ensure you are challenging your hips' strength and mobility in a full 180 degrees of motion.

It's just as important to stress the supporting leg's tension and strength as it is in the leg you are lifting. This tension ensures you are conditioning both legs at the same time for their respective roles while kicking. The supporting leg is providing stability and control while the kicking leg is developing mobility and strength.

You can also adjust this exercise's difficulty by how much support is provided by your upper body. Less upper body support means that your supporting leg needs to work harder to ensure stability. Assistance with the upper body can make it a little bit easier to lift and hold your kicking leg up in the air.

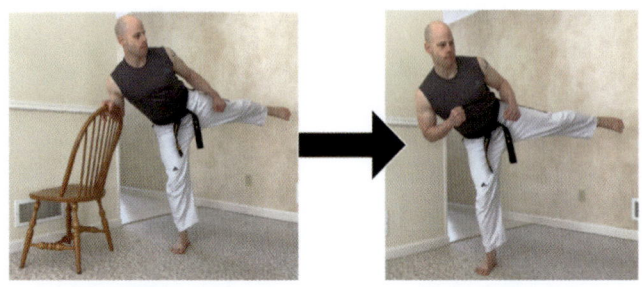

Practicing leg raises without holding onto something is an effective progression for your leg stability and hip strength.

Conditioning exercises

As a martial artist, your best conditioning drills are sparring, bag work, and partner drills. However, some supplemental conditioning can do wonders to improve endurance and explosive power. The following quick exercises are selected because they can easily integrate into a strength training circuit program or some active light recovery on your non-strength training days.

Jumping rope

Skipping rope has long been a staple in boxing, but it isn't as popular in more traditional martial arts training. It's a shame because it's a portable, low-cost form of conditioning that can improve timing, agility, and calf strength.

Air-sits

Jumping is a fantastic conditioning tool. It improves explosive power in the lower body while also testing your cardiovascular endurance. Air-sits are also a great technique to teach you how to pick up your knees in the air if your training demands airborne kicks.

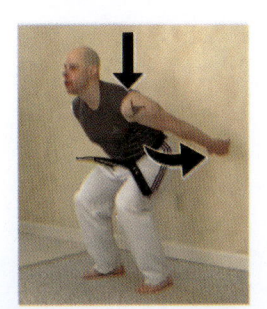

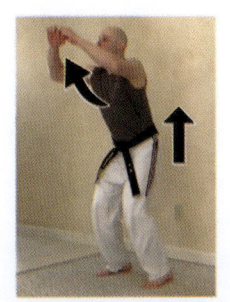

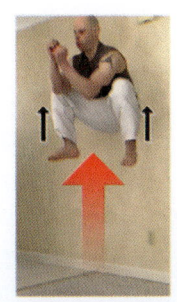

Start sitting your hips back and swing your arms behind you (Left). Extend your legs to jump straight up while swinging your arms upward (Middle). At the peak, tuck your knees up in front of you like you're sitting in a chair.

You can also combine air-sits with burpees where you jump and tuck your knees where you would typically hop up from a push-up position during a burpee. Be sure to land softly and in control to prevent stress on your joints.

Hill Sprints

In my opinion, nothing beats a good hill or even a whole mountain for improving cardiovascular conditioning and leg strength. All you do is start at the bottom of the hill and get to the top as quickly as possible. It's also a lot more rewarding than feeling stuck on a stationary piece of cardio equipment.

Be sure to warm up thoroughly before attempting to run up the hill. Also, take your time as you come down and be careful of your knees. Most injuries and accidents happen while descending an incline rather than going up.

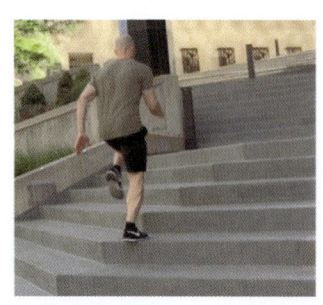

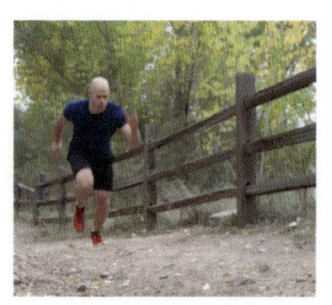

Nothing beats moving your body as fast as you can against the pull of gravity. All you need is a good hill or set of stairs and you're all set!

Chapter 8

Routines for Success

Now that you have a basic understanding of calisthenics exercises for martial arts, it's time to put all of these pieces together into a solid routine. Building a workout routine is like baking a recipe in the kitchen. While each ingredient can hold some value, combining them in a specific plan is the path to results.

Each of the routines in this chapter is designed to help you develop a particular goal, but none of them are static. Consider each one to be a basic template rather than a direct set of instructions. Feel free to experiment and modify them as you see fit.

Here are some basic programming principles to keep in mind to get the most from your training.

#1 Always have a plan

You wouldn't face off against an opponent thinking "I'll just move around and see if anything opens up." That would be crazy! You want to approach your workouts the same way you would an opponent in competition. Have at least some basic idea of what you want to accomplish in each workout.

Sure, your plans can change. As Mike Tyson said, "Everyone has a plan until they get punched in the face." But it's still better to have a plan that you can then change and modify as your situation warrants. Otherwise, you'll risk wasting time and energy doing busy work and being unproductive.

#2 Challenge the capabilities you want to progress

The most basic principle of exercise science is that you gain the functional qualities you challenge. In simplest terms, if you want to get good at doing something then practice doing that very thing. Here's a basic list of useful attributes and how to train for them.

If you want to get stronger, challenge your strength

Building strength requires making your muscles work very hard for a short period, usually around between 3-10 seconds per set. You'll practice anywhere from 2-3 work sets per workout and 1-2 workouts per week.
Keep in mind that your strength is specific to the activity you're performing. For example, doing a hard leg exercise will do little for your grip strength nor will grip work improve your leg strength. This natural law is why it's crucial to know just what sort of strength you want to develop. A sufficient strength-based workout will usually involve a short period of work, (1-5 reps) along with a relatively long rest period usually around 2-5 minutes. These workouts are performed 1-2 times per week.

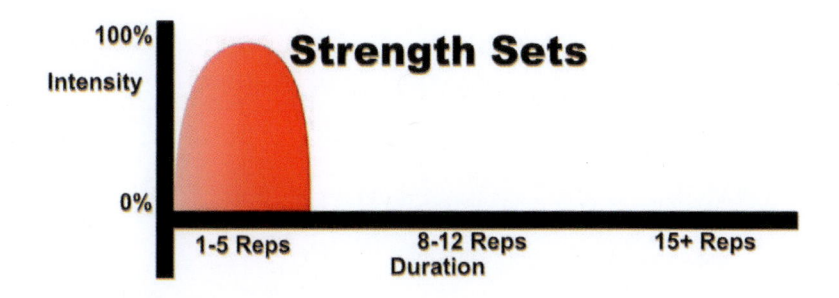

To build stamina, challenge your endurance

Endurance training is on the opposite end of the spectrum where your training durations are relatively long and your rest periods are pretty short. The goal of this sort of training is to challenge your ability to perform as well as possible while under fatigue. You can accomplish this in several ways. You can challenge the stamina of a single muscle group by performing many reps of a single exercise. Doing as many kicks or rows in three minutes is a good example of this sort of training. The other variation is to test your metabolic endurance by stringing several exercises together in a circuit.

Like strength training, endurance training is highly specific to your activity. You may be able to efficiently run ten miles but struggle to last three rounds sparring. This discrepancy is why you want your endurance training to mimic the functional demands of competition so you'll have as much functional carryover as possible.

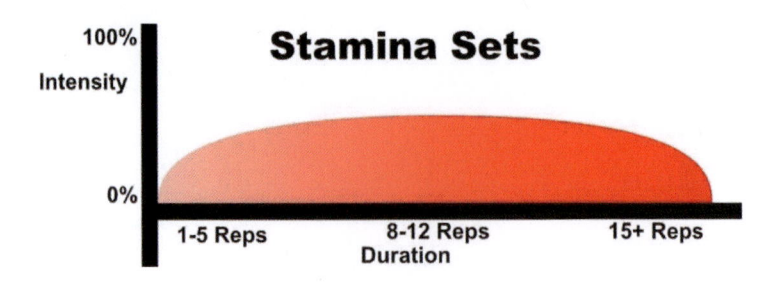

Stamina Sets chart: Intensity 0–100%, Duration 1-5 Reps / 8-12 Reps / 15+ Reps

To become more explosive, challenge your power

Explosive power training is much like strength training where you're attempting to make your muscles use a lot of energy in a short period. It's for this reason you want your explosive training to use low reps (usually between 3-6) with extended rest periods so your neuro-muscular system can remain fresh. Be sure to do your power training early in your workout so your muscles are not tired and you finish before you become very fatigued.

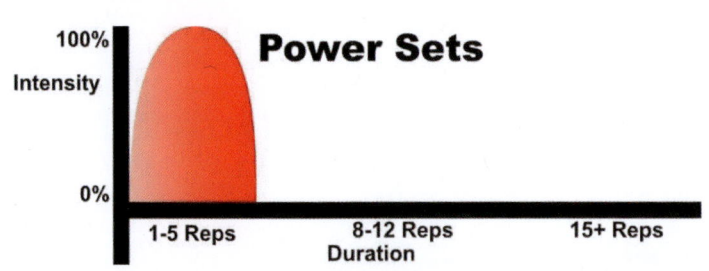

Power Sets chart: Intensity 0–100%, Duration 1-5 Reps / 8-12 Reps / 15+ Reps

Power sets and workouts resemble strength sets in both approach and programming.

To improve balance, challenge your stability

Stability is the foundation of your strength and capability. You cannot be strong, powerful, or fast if you're unstable. The vital importance of stability is why it's crucially important to challenge your stability regularly. Thankfully, the nature of bodyweight training ensures you must create your own total body stability during every exercise. You'll even find the more advanced moves require more stability as you shift your weight around.

You may still want to do some focused stability work, like single-arm or leg training to accelerate your progress especially if you're feeling a little shaky in some positions. If that's the case, practicing standing on one leg or holding a single-arm row on a daily basis can do wonders for helping you feel more grounded.

Stability training is a form of low-fatigue training so it's something you can practice on a very frequent basis which I highly recommend. Doing a little bit every day can help you progress much faster than only working on it once or twice a week.

To improve mobility, work through a greater range of motion

We, martial artists, are no stranger to stretching, but mobility is much more than just passively moving a limb into position. It's also about using the strength of your muscles to control yourself in those positions.

Having control over a broader range of movement gives you the strength and stability to effectively use that range in a functional application. The bigger your useful range is, the more capable you will be. Exercises, like the shifting techniques, build both strength and flexibility which make them an ideal choice for improving mobility.

As with stability work, mobility drills can, and probably should be practiced on a daily basis for maximum benefit.

#3 Keep your routines time and energy efficient

The vast majority of your success as a martial artist comes from your actual martial arts training. All other strength and conditioning work are merely *supplemental*. Understanding this simple lesson can help you keep perspective concerning how much time you should be working out.

I know it can be tempting to include every popular training method under the sun especially when every fitness expert is claiming that their approach is the best. Before you know it, you've incorporated Yoga, Powerlifting, foam rolling, gymnastics, kettlebells, Pilates, primal movement practice, functional training, intervals, variable heart rate training, and plyometric training in your program. If you're lucky, you might even find a few minutes to take a martial arts class!

I recommend focusing on accomplishing just one or two primary objectives in a workout. Doing this will help prevent feature creep from bloating your workouts and diluting the training stimulus. It's also helpful to search for a minimal effective dose in your training. Instead of always trying to do more, aim to do as little work as you can while still gaining a worthwhile benefit.

#4 Set the appropriate frequency

How frequently you train can have a significant influence on your results. Train too often, and you'll burn yourself out. Training too infrequently makes it almost impossible to improve your skills and proficiency.

There are a lot of recommendations out there regarding how frequently you should train, but there is seldom one approach that works for everyone. Some training styles can, and should, be done daily or even multiple times each day. Other methods are best practiced once or twice a week.

There are a lot of variables that can influence the appropriate frequency of exercise, from your diet and sleep habits to even technique. Just keep in mind that you don't have to recover from exercise or training. You only need to recover from *fatigue*, and that can be different from one person to the next. Some people can do 100 push-ups every day and be fine. Others may do half that amount and need a whole week to recover. The simplest way to think about it is training that creates more fatigue requires more rest and therefore less frequency. Workouts that produce less fatigue don't need as much recovery so you can practice them more frequently. Pay attention to how your training makes you feel and adjust your training frequency accordingly.

In general, high-fatigue training, like strength and endurance training should be done 1-3 times a week. Low-fatigue training, like mobility and stability work, can be done 5+ days a week.

#5 Keep a workout log

Adam Savage, from the TV show MythBusters, once stated that the difference between science and just messing around was writing stuff down. This idea is as true in your training as it is with blowing stuff up in the name of science.

I know keeping a log can seem tedious, but using a journal actually saves you time and energy.
Keeping a log gives you structure and focus to your workouts. This aspect alone can save you a ton of energy, not to mention mental stress. Writing down that you're going to do four sets of lunges every Tuesday and Friday ensures that's what you will do with regular consistency.

Aside from structure and clarity, a log also significantly improves your ability to make progress. One of the biggest myths about workout progress is that it will happen if you work hard and put in enough effort. You cannot indefinitely progress by investing more time and energy in your training. Instead, improvement depends on your ability to identify and remember, little windows of opportunity from one workout to the next.

Those windows of opportunity can be notoriously difficult to spot. Sometimes they are big, like adding a couple of reps or trying out an advanced level technique, but most of the time they are much more subtle. Your next improvement could be something like shifting your weight more onto your front heel when practicing lunges, or pulling up your toes during leg raises. Keeping a log helps you stay on the lookout for these little details, so you don't miss them.

Once you do notice some of these windows of opportunity, they won't do you much good if you don't remember them from one workout to the next. Writing them down ensures such details don't slip your mind and you're stuck doing the same workout over and over. Not to mention, that writing down these areas to work on also shows you what to work on when you start your next workout.

#6 Plan your workouts for minimal interference with your martial arts training

The last thing you want is for your conditioning work to interfere with your martial arts practice. The best way to ensure you're not creating an interference affect is to plan your workouts on days you're not doing your martial arts.

Another way to prevent an interference affect is to minimize the fatigue you incur from your conditioning. You can do this in several ways. The first is to cut your training volume. If you're doing five sets, cut it down to 3. If you run for 3 miles cut it down to one. More is not always better when it comes to training, and it's a good idea to experiment and identify what is a minimal effective dose for you.

The other way to cut back on fatigue is to stop each set before reaching muscle failure. If you can do 15 push-ups, finish the set at 10. Every additional rep and moment you spend training costs you exponentially more energy and therefore requires more recovery.

I'm not saying you shouldn't push yourself, you certainly should. I'm just saying you don't have to make each training session a game where you're trying to see how much punishment your body can endure. When you pull back and save energy you recover faster and have minimal interference with your martial arts training while still gaining the benefits you want.

Routine templates

Now that you have the basic principles of routine programming let's take a look at some templates you can use to get started. Feel free to modify these as you see fit.

Warm-up and active recovery routines

These workouts are quick warm-up routines to help you get ready for the day or class ahead. These are also ideal for rest days to speed up recovery and prevent you from getting too stiff the day after a hard training session. These shouldn't create a lot of fatigue so you can practice them most days of the week or even every day if you like.

Complete warm-up

This warm-up routine should cover all of your bases and leave you ready to rock and roll. It's important to not push yourself so hard during this workout to exhaust yourself.

Complete Warm-up

10-20 reps of:
Arm circles,
Torso twists,
Frogger stretch,
Standing knee raises.

Shifting lunges 15 seconds each leg for 2 sets.

Shifting push-ups 20 seconds for 2 sets

Skip lunges 3 reps/leg 2 sets

Front and side raise kicks 1 set of 5 each direction done at moderate speed.

Late for class

This warm-up routine is ideal for when you're short on time and need to get action-ready quickly.

Late For Class

Twisting lunges 10 reps (5/side)

Shifting front-back and side to side push-ups 6 total reps each direction

Skipping with high knees 1 round trip

The morning after

This gentle warm-up is ideal for those times when you're not feeling at your best like when you're tired, stiff, or sore.

> **The Morning After**
>
> Walking high knees with a pause at the top
> 20 total reps
>
> Isometric lunge w/ slow arm circles
> 10-20 reps on each leg.
>
> Slow lying leg raise or knee tuck 5-10 reps
>
> Circle shifting push-ups 3 reps each direction
>
> Rows 6 reps holding the top and bottom stretch position for a few seconds.

Primary workout routines

These routines are the meat and potatoes of your strength and conditioning program. If possible, you should do them on the days you're not practicing your martial arts for optimal recovery. The amount of fatigue they induce can vary, but you'll get the most benefit from exercising these 2-3 times a week on nonconsecutive days.

Full body strength

This plan is a traditional strength and muscle-building routine you can use to build a foundation of power and strength. It begins with a set of shifting push, pull, and lunge movements to warm up your joints and nervous system. The main workout is two supersets with the first focusing on the upper body and the second on the legs and core. Be sure to use the appropriate level of difficulty for each exercise to challenge your muscles within the given number of reps.

Full Body Strength

Warm up:
Shifting push-ups 5-10 reps
Shifting Rows 3-6 reps
Shifting lunges 8-16 reps/ side

1a) Push-ups 3 sets of 8-12 reps
1b) Rows 3 sets of 10-15 reps

2a) Lunges 4 sets of 20-40 reps
2b) Leg Raises 4 sets of 15-30 reps

Explosive power routine

This routine focused on developing pure power and speed. It begins with a light warm-up of the primary exercises you will be practicing. These should be done with a moderate amount of resistance so the required reps shouldn't create much fatigue. One round should be sufficient but include a second warm-up round if you're feeling cold and stiff.

The explosive portion of the workout should help you work up a light sweat without feeling too drained. Try to put as much effort as possible into each rep. If your muscles start to feel heavy on the last set drop it down to 4 or even 3 rounds.

> ## **Explosive Power**
>
> Warm up:
> Light push-ups 4-8 reps
> Light rows 4-8 reps
> Light lunges 8-16 reps
> Light leg raises 5-10 reps
>
> Power sets; 5 rounds of the following:
>
> Explosive push-ups 3 reps
> Explosive Rows 6 reps
> Explosive lunges 6 reps
> Explosive leg raises 9 reps

Power and strength routine

This routine is a combination of power training and strength training. Start off using the same warm-up as the explosive power routine and then perform 2 rounds of explosive sets. Once you're finished with the explosive work move on to the strength portion with 3 rounds of the upper body superset before finishing with the leg and core superset.

> **Power & Strength**
>
> 2 rounds of the following:
> Explosive push-ups 3 reps
> Explosive rows 6 reps
> Jump lunges 6 reps
> Explosive leg raise 9 reps
>
> Perform 3 rounds:
> 1a) Progressive push-ups 6-8 reps
> 1b) Progressive Rows 6-8 reps
>
> 2a) Progressive lunges 20-30 reps
> 2b) Progressive leg raises 15 reps

Muscle endurance routine

This routine is designed to challenge your neuromuscular endurance and mental fortitude. These two qualities are invaluable to any martial artist and can test your resolve to continue fighting when your muscles feel like they are on fire.

You may wish to warm up with 1-2 light sets to get the muscles working and prepare your mind for the pain that's headed your way. Put everything you've got into each set, so your muscles are entirely spent. It's perfectly fine to regress to an easier variation of each exercise as you fatigue to continue doing reps. You can further test your muscles by holding an isometric at the end of each set for 10-15 seconds if you have a high pain tolerance. Give yourself plenty of rest between exercises.

Another interesting variation is to do isometric variations of all of these exercises either as the whole set, or holding an isometric position for 5-10 seconds at the end of each set.

> **Muscle Endurance**
>
> Push-ups:
> As many reps as possible in 3 minutes.
>
> Rows.
> As many reps as possible in 4 minutes.
>
> Explosive lunges
> As many as possible in 2 minutes.
>
> Leg raises
> As many reps as possible in 3.5 minutes.
>
> Skipprope or hill sprints for 5 minutes

Metabolic Endurance Routine

As the saying goes; fatigue makes mice out of all men. Anyone can hit hard and move fast when they are fresh, but things are quite different when the breathing is labored and the heart rate is through the roof. That sort of condition is where many fights are won and lost so it really pays to condition yourself for those circumstances. This routine template will help you do just that.

This routine starts with jumping rope for 5 minutes to warm up. After that, perform the entire circuit moving from one exercise to the next with minimal rest. Use a moderate pace with each set but don't rush through each set and compromise your technique. This isn't a race.

If you're struggling to keep up, add a short rest period (30 seconds should be enough) between each exercise and decrease the break over time.

> ### Metabolic Endurance
>
> Warm up:
> Skip rope for 5 minutes
>
> Perform the following circuit 1-10 times as time and energy warrant.
>
> Explosive lunges 30 reps
> Push-ups 20 reps
> Rows 25 reps
> Leg raises 15 reps
> Shadow boxing 50 punches
> Shadow kicking 30 kicks

Kicking strength routine

This routine is designed to improve your kicking strength and technique. It's also ideal for developing the hip strength and mobility you'll need for groundwork.

Kicking Strength

2 rounds of:
1a) Shifting lunges 10 reps on each side
2b) Alternating leg raises 20 reps

3 rounds of:
2a) Hip raises 10 reps each leg front and back hold up the leg for a 5 count
2b) Lunges 20 reps each leg

Finish with 4 rounds of:
Skip rope 90 seconds 30 seconds rest between sets.

Punching strength routine

This routine will help you target the qualities that are most important for strong and powerful punches.

Punching Strength

Perform 4 sets of the following after a couple of gentle warm-up sets:

Explosive push-ups:
6 reps with 45 seconds rest between sets

Fast rows with towel grip
12 reps 45 seconds rest between sets.

Finish with:
As many push-ups as possible in 90 seconds

As many rows as possible with a towel or handle grip in 2 minutes

Using periodization for long-term progress

There's a saying in fitness that everything works, but nothing works forever. This basically means any routine will initially create a stimulus for change, but all routines eventually plateau as you adapt to that stimulus. A plateau happens to everyone regardless of what sort of routine they practice or how hard they work,

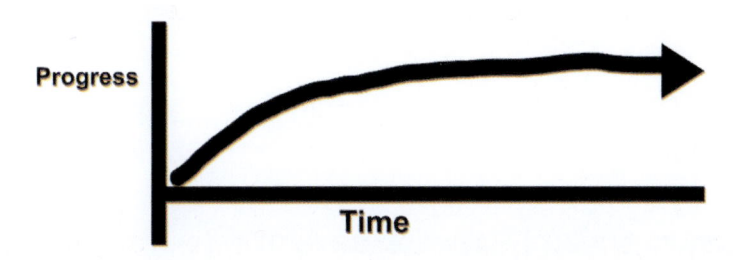

Plateaus can be frustrating, and people react to them in different ways. Some folks become overly frustrated and quit training only to return to it at a later date when their motivation picks back up again. Others resolve to stick to the routine and ride out the plateau with the false hope that it will start to produce results again. Neither of these attitudes will help you make progress in the long term.

Then, you have those who recognize they need to make a change in their training to continue moving forward. This perspective is best, but it can sometimes lead you down unproductive paths. Some athletes adopt a hit and miss approach and select random exercises and workout methods. This approach usually goes hand-in-hand with the false idea that change alone will somehow stimulate the body to keep getting stronger.

The other option is to recognize that you need to adopt a different workout routine. While this is thinking on the right track, you can quickly get lost down numerous rabbit holes as you search for "the best" routine and it's easy to select something at random where, once again, you're hoping to make progress by blind luck and chance.

The practice of periodization helps you avoid all of these scenarios. It gives you a structured plan so you can make productive changes to your routine that help you continue to move forward.

Periodization is merely creating several different workout routines, or "blocks", that you practice at various times throughout the year. Each block emphasizes a functional characteristic like strength or endurance. Your routines may be very similar, but the emphasis on each of your various qualities helps you make more progress than if you tried to work on everything at once throughout the year.

Basic periodization strategies

Here are some basic periodization strategies that you can use as a basic template. Like your workout routine, feel free to use these as a starting point and modify them as you see fit.

Competition periodization

Competitive athletes incorporate a natural periodization plan around their competition seasons. While martial arts competitions are often a year-long practice, it's still a good idea to follow this basic template around your most important competitions throughout the year. Each block can last anywhere from a week or two to a couple of months depending on how much time and energy you need to compete.

Block 1 Offseason

This block is where you're between competitions or seasons. You can now spend a substantial amount of energy in your conditioning workouts, so this is when you want to focus on higher fatigue sessions like muscle endurance and strength-building sessions. You can also use a pretty high frequency for these at about 3-4 times a week.

Block 2 Pre-season

This block is when you're actively getting ready to compete. Most of your energy should now be spent in class and training the specific skills you want to develop to perform at your best. Your strength and conditioning work should downshift into more skill-based shifting and explosive work so the strength and endurance you acquired during the offseason can carry over to your martial arts training.

Block 3 Competition season

During this time, most of your energy should focus on your competitions and preparatory training. Your strength and conditioning workouts are now in maintenance mode as you practice them about twice a week using roughly the same intensities and rep ranges.

Block 4 Postseason

This workout block follows a big competition or sports season. Your body and mind have been pushed to their limit so now is the time for active recovery and any healing if necessary. Some athletes even forego their strength and conditioning sessions at this time and engage in active hobbies like golf or cycling. Your strength sessions shouldn't be taxing during this period and almost feel playful. Now is also an ideal time to identify and work on any weaknesses in preparation for the next offseason training block.

Seasonal periodization

Seasonal periodization is similar to competition periodization only you plan each block around the seasonal changes of Mother Nature. This plan may be ideal if you live in a seasonal environment and find your lifestyle changing with the seasons.

The general idea still applies where you want to plan your resource-intensive training sessions for the seasons you tend to be more sedentary. For example, if you manage to lounge around the house in the winter then use that time for your hard and heavy workouts. If you're more active during the summer months, you can plan workouts that don't require as much time or energy.

Time-based periodization

Some exercise enthusiasts don't have seasonal changes in their lifestyle so opt for a time-based periodization plan. This approach is simple where each block lasts a predetermined amount of time like 4-6 weeks.

Whereas seasonal and competitive periodization may be broken up into 3-4 blocks time-based periodization can include however many blocks you feel fit your needs. Some athletes may use a simple 2-block strategy where they alternate between endurance and strength-focused training. Others may focus on certain skills like wrestling, stand-up fighting, or sparring.

Flexible periodization

Flexible periodization is where you plan out your workouts, but you don't assign each block to a given amount of time or season. This approach works for athletes who find their routine has gone stale in the middle of a block or they feel a routine is still working for them at the end of a block. Instead of planning when you change each block, you stick with a block for as long as you feel you're making progress. You're then free to switch to the next block when you think your current routine has started to get a little long in the tooth.

How to set up your periodization plan

It's easy to feel intimidated by periodization because it means planning out multiple workouts and scheduling them all together. It's much easier to head to the gym and mess around which is why most people do that. But don't worry because here's a simple five-step process that makes it easy to set up your periodization plan.

Step 1 Identify your goals and functional requirements.

As always, a proper plan starts with the end in mind. It's crucially important to get real about what you want to accomplish with your training. Since this is a book about conditioning for martial arts, I'll assume you want to become a better martial artist.

Once you have your goal in place, write out a few of the essential functional qualities that will help you accomplish that goal. These qualities can include building strength and endurance, but it can also involve personal objectives like improving kicking strength or stamina for sparring. Whatever you need, write those down for what you'll focus on for each block.

> **Goal:**
> Advance to blue belt in June
>
> **Qualities:**
> Stronger kicks
> Endurance when rolling
> Upper body strength

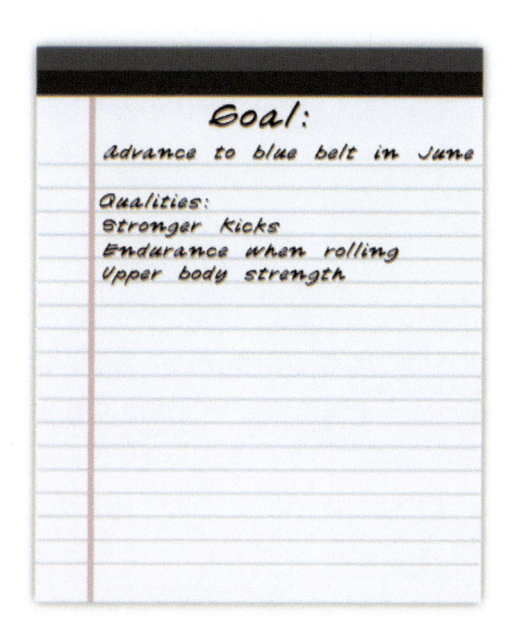

Step 2 Identify your blocks and timeframes

The next step is to plan your workout block timeframes. Are you going to design around a big competition? Maybe seasonal blocks are the way to go. Be sure to plan your blocks, so they correspond to the number of objectives you listed in step 1.

> **Goal:**
> advance to blue belt in June
>
> Qualities:
> Stronger Kicks
> Endurance when rolling
> Upper body strength
>
> Block #1 6-Weeks
> Focus on Upper body strength
>
> Block #2 6-Weeks
> Focus on kicking
>
> Block #3 4-Weeks
> Focus on rolling/ endurance

Step 3 Write out a weekly plan for each block.

Now that you have your block time frame and objectives it's time to plan your weekly routine for each block. I recommend just starting with a basic routine outline for the week where you plan your training days and what you'll practice each day.

Strength Block

Monday Strength Workout	Tuesday Judo Class
Wednesday Rest Day	Thursday Strength Workout
Friday Kick Boxing	Saturday Strength Workout
Sunday Rest Day	

Step 4 Write out your routine for each workout.

Lastly, plan each workout including what exercises you'll practice and how you'll apply them.

Strength Workout — Monday

Warm up:
3 minutes skipping rope

Push-Ups:
1-2 light sets of incline push-ups. 10-20 reps each

3 work sets close push-ups 3-5 reps

Rows:
1-2 light sets of table rows to warm up 8-12 reps

3 work sets of single arm table rows. 5 reps/side

Strength Workout — Thursday

Warm up:
3 minutes skipping rope

Lunges:
1 minute alternating spot lunges

Walking twisting lunges
5 sets of 45 seconds

Leg raises:
1-2 light sets of lying knee raises 8-15 reps

3 work sets of hanging knee raise 15-20 reps

I recommend using a simple Google Docs or Sheets file for each workout block and keeping all of your workouts in a single folder on your Google Drive. That way, you have access to all of your workouts on any digital device, and you can modify them as needed.

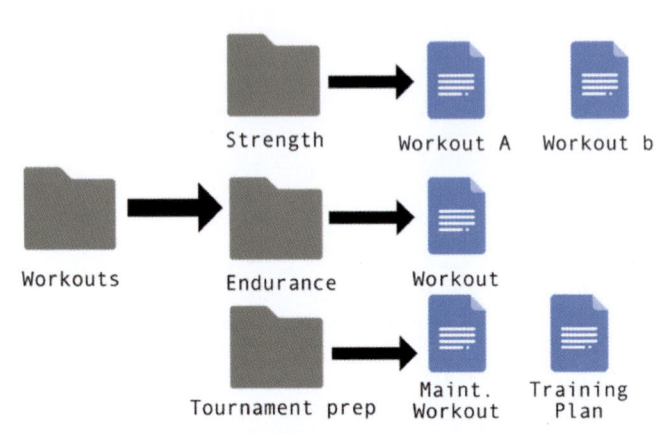

Keeping your workouts in a simple digital format helps you stay organized.

If you prefer an analog setup, you can use a separate notebook for each workout or place a different workout for each section in one of those multiple subject notebooks.

Most training blocks change over with changes in season or life events, like the end of a sports season. Sometimes a block can last a seemingly random amount of time like 3 weeks or 12 workouts. This can be a little more difficult to track and know when to change to the next block.

I recommend setting up a reminder in your calendar so it will pop up at the end of each block. That way, you don't have to track or count weeks or workouts.

Step 5 Apply and modify.

Don't worry too much about getting your plan or workouts perfect at first. It's impossible to know what you need and what's going to work best especially when you're starting. I know it can be tempting to endlessly research your plan to make it as effective as possible but this can be a big mistake. Too much "research" can easily lead to paralysis by analysis and second-guessing every detail to the point where you get stuck and never take action.

You'll learn more about what works best for you once you start applying your workouts and making notes about how things are going for you. You can then modify your workouts and even your whole periodization plan through experience. Trial and error are why many professional athletes can take a few seasons to dial in their program and figure out what works best for them. So don't feel like you have to stick to a given plan if something's not working for you, but also don't change your program so much that you compromise the structure of your plan. Adjust, modify, and get dialed in. It won't take long before you've created a custom plan that's perfect for you.

Chapter 9

How to Be Action-Ready At All Times

One of the most vexing challenges martial artists face is how to be physically ready to fight without a thorough warm-up. As a Taekwon-Do practitioner, I've heard plenty of criticism about how the signature kicks of the discipline wouldn't be practical for self-defense. After all, what good is a high kick if you can't throw it in a surprise attack?

It's not practical to only be physically capable after a lengthy warm-up. This is true for both self-defense and general health. You should feel light, fast, and ready to move most of the time even on days you don't exercise. Feeling stiff and slow shouldn't be one's normal state.

Staying action-ready isn't just about being able to move when trouble goes down. It also means maintaining a physical and mental state where you can comfortably move and use your body throughout the day. It helps to reduce stress on your joints, eases muscle stiffness, and decreases the risk of injury when working. It is the natural state you were meant to be in before the artificial influences of chairs, desks and TV came into your life. You don't have to shun modern living to be action-ready either. All you need is a few of the following techniques.

Action-ready exercises

Being action-ready requires practicing light movements and exercises every single day or even multiple times every day if possible. As you can imagine, this would be almost impossible to do if you always had to rely on using a piece of equipment that anchors your physical activity to a specific time and place. The unrestricted freedom to train anywhere at any time is yet another advantage of bodyweight training.

#1 Arm and shoulder circles

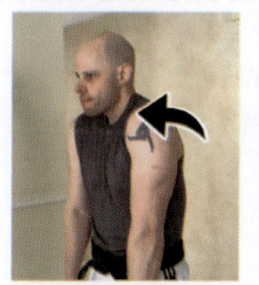

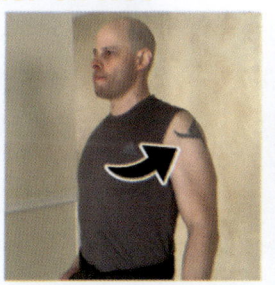

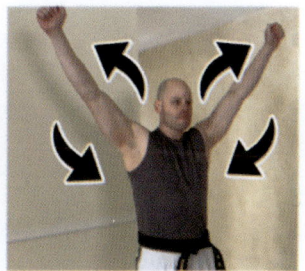

Moving your shoulders and arms in big controlled circles does wonders for your back and shoulder health.

The simple act of moving your arms in a big stretched-out circle helps to lube your shoulder joints while improving the strength and stability of your shoulder and torso muscles. You can also circle your shoulders to emphasize the mobility and tension control of your chest and back.

These simple movements improve muscle tone, decrease neck strain, stretch your back and open up your chest for easier breathing.

The key is to stretch your arms as far out as you can with each rotation. Try to draw the biggest circle possible with each arm. You may find it helpful to do one arm or shoulder at a time if you feel it uncomfortable to use both arms at once. Be sure to circle your arms and shoulders in both directions.

#2 Front and back handclasp

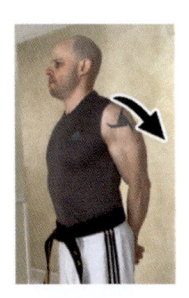

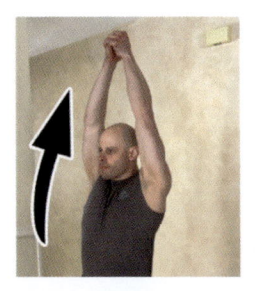

These two exercises have an almost miraculous therapeutic effect for loosening tight muscles while strengthening weak ones in the upper back and shoulders. The behind-the-back handclasp is done by clasping your fingers together and trying to squeeze your arms behind you using the muscles in your back. Don't worry if you can barely touch your fingertips at first. Your mobility and strength will improve quickly.

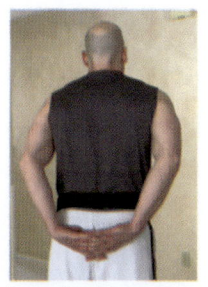

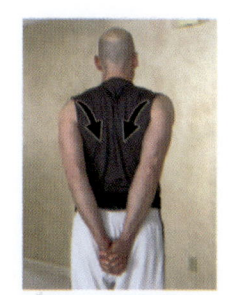

You may find your hands stay open and your shoulders are apart when you first do this. Keep practicing every day and your back will grow stronger pulling your arms and hands closer together.

The front raise hand clasp involves placing your hands in front of you and then lifting them in front and overhead as high as you can. This technique is one of the best ways to loosen up stiff shoulders and tight lats.

With both of these exercises, try your best to keep your spine straight and avoid arching backward to achieve more range of motion with the arms.

#3 Standing hip and ankle circles

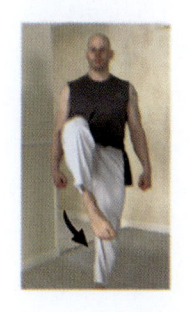

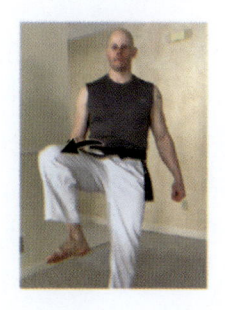

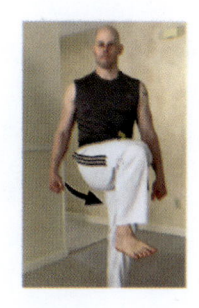

Standing on one leg is the white belt level of lunges but it's also a great daily action-ready exercise. Circling your hip and ankle joint improves mobility and dexterity plus your stability and coordination as well.

#4 Forward bend

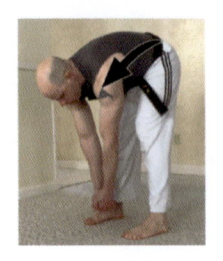

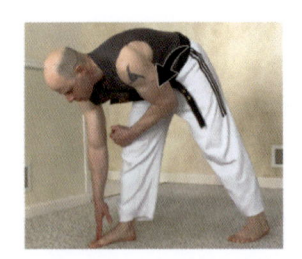

The forward bend is a natural posterior chain stretch that can loosen up tight muscles in your back and hamstrings.

You don't always have to do this exercise as the classic bend over and touch your toes. You can also practice this with one foot in front of the other to emphasize one leg and work on specific muscles on each side of your body.

This exercise is also easy to incorporate throughout your day if you ever need to bend over to pick up something light off the floor.

#5 Torso twist

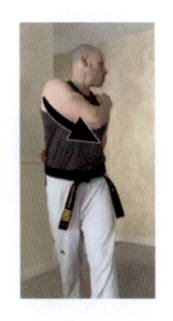

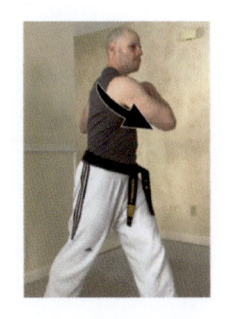

Twisting your body is a great way to condition and mobilize the muscles that run along your spine. You can practice this twisting motion in several ways. The first is to place one hand behind you and the other hand on top of your shoulder and then gently twist and hold toward your back arm.

Another variation is more dynamic as you lift your arms slightly and twist from one side to the other in a smooth movement. Be sure to allow the heel of your back foot to come off the floor to relieve any twisting stress on the knee.

#6 Shifting lunges or squats

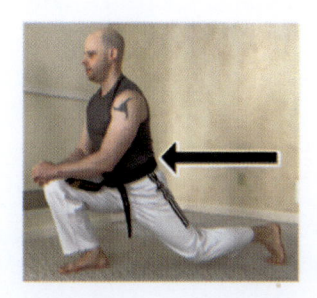

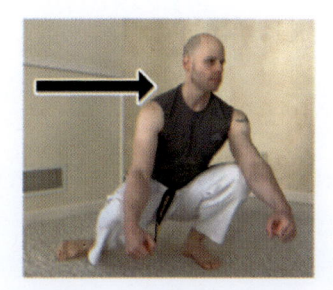

Shifting lunges or squats are a fantastic exercise to keep your lower body action-ready. Granted, their practice depends on what sort of clothing you may be wearing as this can be difficult in more formal attire. Nonetheless, taking a few moments each day to squat down and move around a bit can do a lot for your mobility and stability and keep your lower body ready for almost anything.

I know these techniques don't seem too difficult, and that's precisely why they are so useful. They are not meant to be something that causes you to work very hard or break a sweat. You don't even need to follow any particular routine to practice them. Just take advantage of them anytime you've been sitting for a while or are feeling a little stiff and sluggish.

Conclusion

Well, my friend, it's time for me to bow out and let you apply what you have learned. While this is the end of the book, I still have a lot more valuable information to share with you. I invite you to check out over 1,000 free videos on the Red Delta Project YouTube channel and the in-depth Red Delta Project Podcast. If you have any specific ideas or questions feel free to send them my way at reddeltaproject@gmail.com, or you can DM me via Instagram @red.delta.project.

I wish you the best of luck in your training and continued growth both as an athlete and a martial artist.

- Matt Schifferle